- **What are antioxidants and why should you care about them?**

- **Can folic acid help prevent heart disease and birth defects?**

- **What's the difference between soluble and insoluble fiber?**

- **What's so special about olive oil, anyway?**

"It seems like every week we read something different about what we should eat. It can get really confusing—and frustrating.

"Public understanding of science should not come down to who or what sounds most convincing. But our national fixation with quick-fix solutions encourages and embraces this approach. My approach to science takes the important details into account and places them in a context that's easier to understand. When food and nutrition news breaks, I am there to serve as translator. Knowledge is a form of empowerment and I am intent on passing my knowledge on to you."

—from the Introduction by Dr. Ed Blonz

POWER NUTRITION

How to Live Longer,
Prevent Illness,
and Be Healthier with
Good Nutrition

Dr. Ed Blonz

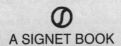

A SIGNET BOOK

SIGNET
Published by the Penguin Group
Penguin Putnam Inc., 375 Hudson Street,
New York, New York 10014, U.S.A.
Penguin Books Ltd, 27 Wrights Lane,
London W8 5TZ, England
Penguin Books Australia Ltd, Ringwood,
Victoria, Australia
Penguin Books Canada Ltd, 10 Alcorn Avenue,
Toronto, Ontario, Canada M4V 3B2
Penguin Books (N.Z.) Ltd, 182–190 Wairau Road,
Auckland 10, New Zealand

Penguin Books Ltd, Registered Offices:
Harmondsworth, Middlesex, England

First published by Signet, an imprint of Dutton NAL,
a member of Penguin Putnam Inc.

First Printing, October, 1998
10 9 8 7 6 5 4 3 2 1

A Note to the Reader
The ideas, procedures, and suggestions contained in this book are not intended as a substitute for medical treatment by a physician. The reader should regularly consult a physician in matters relating to health.

 REGISTERED TRADEMARK—MARCA REGISTRADA

Printed in the United States of America

Contents

Introduction

The Power Is in Your Hands

Do you want to understand the power that nutrition has over heart disease, cancer, and long life? What are anti-oxidants and why should you care about them? What makes a food "unsafe" to eat? Do you want to know how food affects your mood and what food processing does to foods? Did you know that some saturated fats are OK? But which ones? And what's so special about olive oil? Can folic acid affect heart disease and birth defects? What are free radicals, and are they always dangerous? What's the difference between soluble and insoluble fiber? When is risk not that risky?

. . . And what about complex carbohydrates, phyto-chemicals, protein, allergies, benevolent bugs, olestra, pesticides, biotechnology, food additives, and glycemic indexes?

There is a lot of information out there, but what does it all mean? *Power Nutrition* has your answer.

In this book I will answer these and many other important questions about foods, nutrition, and health. I will explain what "good nutrition" is all about, and in the process you will find out what it takes to live longer in better health.

What makes this book different from others is that I will

spell it all out in a way that helps you understand "why." In addition to telling you which foods can affect your moods or what foods help to lower your risk of heart disease, cancer, or diabetes, I explain how it all works. After reading this book, you will understand what's in food, how it's processed, which foods you need to be eating and which ones you should avoid. You will possess the information you need to help you to live longer in better health because you will have the power of food working for you and not against you.

Power Nutrition: The name says it all.

Your Future Begins Now

According to the National Center for Health Statistics, more than 62 million people are diagnosed with some form of heart disease in a typical year; 40 million of these people will be less than sixty-five years of age. One out of every two Americans is at risk for developing cardiovascular disease sometime during their lifetime. Although it's desirable to have a cholesterol level less than 200 mg/dl, at present 96 million adults have cholesterol levels 200 and higher, with 37 million having levels of 240 or more. Every year, about 42 percent of all deaths are due to heart disease.

Only 19 percent of adults are within their ideal weight range, while 76 percent of men and 60 percent of women are clinically overweight. Even more sobering is the fact that obesity is on the rise among our nation's youth.

Fifty million Americans aged six and older have high-blood pressure. More than twenty-five million Americans suffer from osteoporosis; about five million of them are men. Sixteen million Americans have some form of diabetes, with an estimated eight million cases as yet undiagnosed. Insulin-dependent (type 1) diabetes accounts for 10 percent of all cases, while non-insulin-dependent (type 2) diabetes accounts for the rest. The incidence of type-2 diabetes, which is often related to obesity, has more than doubled since 1958.

The news on cancer is not much better. More than ten million Americans are living with some form of cancer. It is now estimated that some half-a-million people will die of cancer this year—that's more than 1,500 a day. These are all shocking statistics.

Why Aren't We Doing Better?

One explanation is that there is an imposing gap between scientific research and public understanding. These days, information about foods, nutrition, and health comes at us from all sides through the printed and electronic media, advertisements, food labels, and now, the Internet. With the popular press often playing up the most headline-grabbing aspect of a study, it's no wonder that the public is left wondering what it all means. What you hear or read about is often biased by commercial interests—someone trying to sell you something. The bottom line is that it is difficult to cope, let alone decide what's best for you or your family. As a result, we end up grasping at the straws of quick-fix formulas and magic-bullet cures.

It is my mission in this book to help you bridge the gap and cut through the confusion on a wide range of food, nutrition, and health issues. You will read the story behind the story and understand how it can all fit into your daily life. I include topics you want to know about, such as fats, food safety, fiber, food additives, vitamin supplements, phytochemicals, and nutrition and aging. I spell out the science in a way that eliminates rather than contributes to your confusion.

- For example, we keep hearing how "low fat" or "no fat" are the only passports to good health, so many of us are rightfully puzzled when we learn that other cultures seem able to feast on high-fat diets while still enjoying good health and long life. The French, for example, are known for their rich cuisine, yet their rate of heart disease is among the lowest of all developed countries. If you look to Greece and Italy, you find a Mediterranean diet, where good health goes along with a generous intake of olive oil. After I explain how high-fat diets work in these cultures, you will better understand why they haven't been working for you.

- The average age in this country continues to climb, and the first of the baby-boomer generation have now reached the half-century mark. Many are confused about nutrition's special powers to combat the aging process. When we are younger, we feel immune and detached from the process of aging. Life, however, is a cumulative process, and health in our later years reflects our earlier habits. *Power Nutrition* gives you a simple understanding of how the body's metabolism changes and which nutrients are especially important for long-term health. You will learn about food supplements, phytochemicals, and changing eating habits. I will give you strategies for how to increase good health in later life.

- Salt will never be a health food, but only a minority need worry about salt in their diets. Yet many people unnecessarily select bland, salt-free foods only because they are mistakenly told that it's better for their health. I explain what salt does in the body and why it's added to foods. After reading this section you'll know how to find out if salt is likely to be a problem for you, and you'll be aware of where it is in our food supply.

Why Listen to Me?

It seems like every week we read something different about what we should eat. It can get really confusing—and frustrating. I realized early on in my career as a nutrition scientist that I had a special ability to translate complex scientific concepts into a language that people could understand. Rather than suffer on the sidelines, I decided to become a full-time "communicator" and I began writing a weekly column on nutrition and health for my local newspaper. Since that time, my weekly column has grown in popularity and it's now nationally syndicated, going out to more than six hundred papers around the country. I receive myriad questions from readers on foods, food science, nutrition, and health, and I answer them in my columns. This gives me a good understanding of what people want to know and where they are confused.

As a working journalist, I also receive press packets on foods and nutrition-related topics. This information often serves as fodder for the stories you read and hear about. Many of the packets, unfortunately, are long on spin and short on science—most of the ink going toward the sales job. Today's media are littered with a rapid succession of quick-take stories. This is unfortunate, for not all science fares well when force-distilled down to a headline and a few paragraphs. Critical details are ignored and research conclusions get taken out of context.

Public understanding of science should not come down to who or what sounds most convincing. But our national fixation with quick-fix solutions encourages and embraces this approach. My approach to science takes the important details into account and places them in a context that's easier to understand. When food and nutrition news breaks, I am there to serve as translator. Knowledge is a form of empowerment, and I am intent on passing my knowledge on to you.

The Power Is Yours for the Taking

Food should be one of life's greatest pleasures. But in today's sound-bite society we have come to focus more on what we shouldn't be eating than on what we should. We spend our time traipsing from one food fear to the next—all the time obsessing about the excess fat in our diet. I want to help you develop your ability to separate fact from fiction so that you can better understand the relationship between food and health.

After reading *Power Nutrition*, you will feel the yoke of scientific oppression lifted from your shoulders as well as your dining table. You will gain a new appreciation for everything that good foods and nutrition can bring to your life.

PART I

Understanding the Basics of a Balanced Diet

1. Protein:

It's What We're Made Of

Protein is a key ingredient in every cell of the body. It is needed to make hair, skin, nails, muscles, organs, blood cells, nerve, bone and brain tissue, enzymes, hormones, antibodies, chemical messengers, and the DNA and RNA used to form the genetic code of life. That's quite a lineup! Perhaps that's why the word *protein* comes from the Greek *proteos,* which means "of prime importance."

All the proteins in our body share the same basic structure, in that they are all made from building blocks called amino acids. There are many different types of protein, but only about twenty-two kinds of amino acids. Of these twenty-two, our body can manufacture all but nine. The reason we need protein in our diet is to supply these nine "essential" amino-acid building blocks.

Proteins tend to be large molecules, and in most cases they are much too large to be absorbed intact. During digestion, the body utilizes specialized digestive enzymes to separate dietary proteins into their individual amino acids. Only then can they be absorbed and used by the body as raw materials to make the variety of proteins necessary for good health.

In the developing countries of Africa, Asia, and South America, protein foods tend to be scarce, and deficiencies are not only present, they can be life-threatening. For generally well-nourished people, a protein intake below required levels will not pose problems if it's only for a day or two now and then. But if the body consistently fails to get enough protein, it will begin showing signs of deficiency.

Depending on the length and degree, symptoms of an ongoing protein deficiency could include: increased susceptibility to disease, fatigue, anemia, hair and skin problems, mental confusion, pallor, digestive disturbances, muscle wasting, weight loss, and eventually death.

But as essential as protein is, eating too much on a regular basis is also not wise—and in the United States, overconsumption is the norm, not the exception. First of all, the average individual does *not* benefit from extra protein, mainly because there is no way to store it for later use. When overindulged with this relatively expensive food, the body, for the most part, has no option but to turn it into body fat. This conversion places an extra demand on the liver and kidneys, the two organs responsible for converting excess amino acids into fat.

There is also some data that having too much protein contributes to the risk of osteoporosis. This occurs because the processing of excess amino acids can effectively drain calcium from the body. The idea, then, is to have enough, but not too much.

How Much Protein Do You Need?

One way to estimate your daily protein requirement is to count 11 grams of protein for every 30 pounds of body weight. By this method, a 150-pound adult needs about 55 grams of protein per day. (Note: If you're overweight, use the ideal body weight for someone of your height.) Those over sixty years of age should count about 15 grams of protein per 30 pounds of body weight.

Pregnant women should add an extra 10 grams of protein per day, and nursing mothers an extra 12 to 15 grams during the first six months. Growing children require more protein in relation to their body weight: about ¹/₂ gram of dietary protein per pound from age one up to age fourteen.

Understanding what a gram of protein is can be confusing. The following examples of the protein content of some typical foods should give you some perspective:

Meat and Dairy Proteins	
1 large egg	.6 g
1 oz. cheddar/jack/Swiss cheese	.7 g
4 oz. hamburger patty	.28 g
8 oz. steak	.69 g
4 oz. fish (trout)	.30 g
4 oz. roast chicken breast	.34 g
1 cup low-fat milk	.9 g
1 cup fruit yogurt	.10 g

Meatless Goes Mainstream

About 12.4 million Americans consider themselves vegetarians, according to a *Time*/CNN survey, and their numbers are continuing to grow. According to another poll, conducted for the magazine *Vegetarian Times,* almost half the vegetarians said they made the change for health reasons. For others, vegetarianism resulted from beliefs about animal welfare, the influence of family or friends, concern for the environment, religious convictions, or other ethical concerns.

> But the mere fact that one's entire diet is based on grains, vegetables, and fruits is not an automatic passport to long life and well-being. Balance, variety, and moderation are the keys to good nutrition whether or not meat appears on your plate. After all, french fries, chips, and doughnuts *are* vegetarian foods.

Because of its focus on fruits, vegetables, and grains, however, the health potential of a vegetarian diet is impressive. Health statistics for vegetarians include lower rates of heart disease, obesity, obesity-related diabetes, colon cancer, lung cancer, breast cancer, hypertension, osteoporosis, kidney stones, gallstones, and diverticular disease. Such findings explain why nearly all health professionals recommend a diet focused on nutrient-rich, high-fiber plant foods.

Although a vegetarian, by definition, is one who eschews all foods of animal origin, we're now seeing a variety of new categories under the vegetarian umbrella.

- *Vegan* (also called strict vegetarian): Consumes no foods of animal origin (no dairy products).
- *Lacto vegetarian:* The only animal products consumed are dairy.
- *Ovo vegetarian:* The only animal products eaten are eggs.
- *Lacto-ovo vegetarian:* The only animal products eaten are dairy and eggs.
- *Pesco vegetarian:* Fish is the only animal product consumed.
- *Pollo vegetarian:* Chicken is the only animal product consumed.
- *Semi-vegetarian:* Meat, fish, or poultry are eaten, but only occasionally.

To have a healthy vegetarian diet, it's important to understand the fundamentals of good nutrition. Most foods have some amino acids. Animal proteins, such as meat, fish, eggs, and dairy products, are *complete* proteins because they contain all the essential amino acids (EAAs). Except for soybeans, vegetable proteins such as grains and legumes are *incomplete* proteins because they lack one or more EAAs. You can easily meet your daily protein requirement by eating only vegetable proteins, however, by combining different foods so that sufficient amounts of all the EAAs are consumed.

In terms of their EAA profile, there are three basic types of vegetable protein: *whole grains,* such as rice, corn, oats, and barley; *legumes,* such as beans and lentils; and *nuts and seeds,* such as almonds and peanuts, and sunflower and sesame seeds. By planning your meals to include foods from two or more of these groups, you end up creating a complete protein. For example, by eating both rice (grains) and beans (legumes), you supply the body with the daily EAAs it needs. This type of "complementary protein" combining is the essence of vegetarianism.

At one time, we thought that the body needed all the EAAs to be consumed at the same meal. Recently, however, scientists have determined that the body can successfully make protein so long as the full complement of EAAs is eaten over the course of a day.

A strict vegetarian diet can provide all but two of the vitamins you need. *Vitamin B_{12},* needed for red blood cells and nerve tissue, is only found in bacteria and animal foods. Vegetarians can use specially fermented soy products, such as tempeh or miso, as a dietary source. The alternative is to rely on foods fortified with vitamin B_{12} or a food supplement.

Vitamin D, needed for calcium absorption and bone formation, is found in fish and vitamin D-fortified milk products. In addition, the body produces this nutrient upon exposure to direct sunlight. Again, the alternative is to rely on a fortified food or a food supplement.

The decision to go vegetarian should not be looked upon as giving something up, but rather as a change in approach to eating. In our society, being a vegetarian is perceived by some as difficult. But that's not the body talking; that's our meat-minded culture. Any move away from the dietary mainstream takes conviction, but you don't have to sign a lifetime contract. The vegetarian experience can open up a new world of ingredients, tastes, and methods of food preparation that can have positive health benefits whether it's for one or two days a week, or a lifetime.

Vegetarian Proteins	
1 oz. (20–30) almonds	6 g
1 cup tofu	18 g
1 cup cooked lentils	18 g
1 cup white rice	6 g
1 cup cooked pasta (no sauce)	7 g
1/2 cup kidney beans	8 g
2 tbsp. peanut butter	8 g
1 cup cooked corn	5 g
1 slice sandwich bread	2 g
1 cup broccoli	3 g

Do Athletes Need More Protein?

The nutritional needs of an athlete, or any physically active individual, can be broken into two categories: supplying raw materials for building muscles and providing energy for the muscles to perform. Although at one time it was thought that the only food for an athlete was a thick steak, nutrition for athletes has grown into a sophisticated branch of science, complete with research journals and sports laboratories around the world. Today we continue to learn how nutrients affect performance, whether it's a daily walk, riding a bicycle, pumping iron at the local gym, or running down the football field.

It's now believed that intensive muscle building or endurance events can as much as double the body's protein requirement. But since the typical diet already contains twice the protein the body needs, there's rarely a need to add protein.

Like anyone else, when athletes take in more protein than their body needs, the excess is changed into energy, and that usually means fat. That process, though, can cause problems for an athlete in training. Converting protein to energy places a load on the kidneys, the organ responsible for removing the unused protein waste from the body. Excess protein can also cause a loss of dietary calcium.

Nonetheless, protein-powder supplements that promise dramatic results and bulging muscles continue to sell well at gyms and health-food stores. Remember, it's the exercise, not the excess protein, that builds muscles.

2. Dietary Fat

Fat, a member of the lipid family, is the most concentrated source of energy in living things; it contains over twice the calories (energy) of protein or carbohydrates. Because we need to be mobile, our body is designed to turn virtually all excess dietary energy into fat and store it as an energy reserve.

Fat provides insulation for the body and padding around sensitive internal organs. Several nutrients are found in the fat portion of our foods, including vitamins A, E and K, the essential fatty acids, and many important phytochemicals. When eaten, fats slow the rate at which the stomach empties, causing a feeling of fullness and satisfaction. You may be surprised to learn that there's nothing inherently "wrong" with fat. Indeed, for most people, fats provide some of the most wonderful tastes and textures to our food.

Let's take a closer look at all the key players in the fat saga.

Fat's Ins and Outs

The terms "fat" and "oil" tend to be used interchangeably. The main difference between them is that fats are solid at room temperature, and oils are liquid. For the sake of clarity, I will be using the generic term "fat" throughout. There are three basic types of fat: saturated, monounsaturated, and polyunsaturated.

Saturated fat is found primarily in animal products, such as butter, lard, eggs, meat, and poultry. Vegetable sources of saturated fat include coconut oil, palm oil, palm-kernel oil, and cocoa butter.

Monounsaturated fat is found in different quantities in most vegetable oils, some of which are primarily mono-unsaturated; these include canola (rapeseed), olive, almond, avocado, and peanut oils.

Polyunsaturated fat is found in the oils of seeds and some nuts, including corn, soy, safflower, sesame, and walnut. Polyunsaturated fat is the only type known to be required by the body. Fish oils are unique in the animal world because they contain polyunsaturated fat as well as saturated.

Cholesterol

There's often confusion over the relative roles of fat and cholesterol. Cholesterol is not the same as fat, but they both belong to the lipid family. Cholesterol is a waxy, fat-like substance with a complex structure resembling honeycomb. Unlike fat, the body does not use cholesterol for energy; this complex compound is an essential structural element in every cell of the body. In addition, cholesterol is a raw material for a number of hormones, including estrogen and testosterone.

Dietary cholesterol can only be found in foods of animal origin, and it's the same as the cholesterol in your blood. But there the similarity ends. Every milligram of cholesterol in your food does not end up cruising around in your bloodstream. In fact, the body's ability to absorb dietary cholesterol decreases as the level in your diet goes up. Most of the cholesterol in the bloodstream, it turns out, is manufactured by the liver as it's needed; when cholesterol is absorbed from the foods we eat, the liver is programmed to make less. In some people, however, this coordination malfunctions. These individuals have to pay special attention to the level of fat and cholesterol in their diets.

Triglycerides

For simplicity, you could almost use the terms *fats* and *triglycerides* interchangeably. A triglyceride is the way that nature bundles fats together, including fats in the diet, in the bloodstream, and even those fats in the body's energy storage depots. Triglycerides look like a squat letter *E,* the three prongs representing the individual saturated or unsaturated fats that make up the triglyceride.

The level of triglycerides in the bloodstream usually goes up after eating, even if there's a limited amount of fat in the meal. That's because the body is programmed to convert most excess protein or carbohydrates into triglycerides, the energy form best suited for storage. A high intake of alcohol or sugars such as fructose, sucrose, or glucose also increases blood triglyceride levels. Not much is known about how an elevated triglyceride level impacts health. In general, people with high triglycerides tend to have a higher risk of heart disease, but it's unclear what role, if any, triglycerides play. Suffice it to say, any abnormal readings should be closely monitored.

Our Fat Transport System

Because triglycerides and cholesterol cannot dissolve in the body's water-based blood, they have to be shuttled through the body inside carriers called lipoproteins. As regards the level of cholesterol in the blood, there are two distinct cholesterol carriers that are of interest. The first, called *low-density lipoprotein (LDL),* can be thought of as the carrier of cholesterol as it goes into the general circulation. The second, called *high-density lipoprotein (HDL),* shuttles the cholesterol on its way out of the body. As the proportion of blood cholesterol traveling in the LDLs goes up, so does your risk of heart disease. By contrast, as the cholesterol in the HDLs goes up, your risk decreases. It's convenient to think of LDLs as the "least desirable" and HDLs as the "highly desirable" forms of cholesterol.

Which Fats Are Best?

Over the past decade, unsaturated fats have mistakenly been given a clean slate while saturated fats were viewed as the unmitigated problem child of the fat family. Recent research, however, points to a need to change this particular good fat/bad fat approach.

Saturated fats have indeed been associated with an increased level of LDL cholesterol, but not all saturated fats have the same cholesterol-raising effect. Stearic acid, a saturated fat found in cocoa butter (chocolate), and some animal fats (beef tallow), have been shown to have little effect on one's blood cholesterol level. If consumed as part of a balanced diet, even the saturated tropical oils—coconut, palm, and palm-kernel—are not the dietary demons they once were thought to be.

Polyunsaturated oils, once touted for their cholesterol-lowering ability, were long thought to be the ideal fat. Recent research, however, has linked an elevated intake of polyunsaturates with undesirable side effects such as suppression of the immune system, increased risk of cancer, and gallstone formation.

Then there's one type of fat that should be either completely avoided or kept to an absolute minimum. This is processed fats, called partially hydrogenated fats, which are used to make margarine, shortening, and many processed foods. Partially hydrogenated fats are discussed later in this chapter.

Monounsaturated oils are the only category of fats that

continue to receive a clean bill of health. As such, these should remain the focus of your diet.

Is a Low-Fat Diet Important?

Scientific research has found a strong association between the amount of fat consumed and the risk of developing heart disease and cancer. But notice that word *association*. There are also associations between those killer diseases and physical inactivity, stress, smoking, high blood pressure, obesity, and low fiber intake. Your level of risk also depends on whether the disease runs in your family.

> An important point lost in all today's antifat furor is that if you eat a well-balanced, high-fiber diet, don't smoke, have normal blood pressure and weight and an active, stress-free lifestyle, the "riskiness" of your fat intake shrinks dramatically.

So why do we pick on fat? One reason is that we can eat only so many Calories in a day. Because fat is such a concentrated energy source, too much fat means too little of the other foods we need. A lack of these other foods—fruits, vegetables, and grains—deprives the body of the nutrients and fiber needed to remain healthy.

Another reason is connected with the fact that fats have a nasty habit of changing into *"free radicals"*—reactive compounds that can damage the cells in the body in a way that leads to heart disease, cancer, and other degenerative diseases. The body gets most of its energy when fats combine with oxygen inside the energy-producing compartment of the cell. Fats and cholesterol, however, have a nasty ability to react with oxygen in the wrong places. When this happens, they don't release energy. Rather, they become "oxidized" and change into free radicals. The higher the fat consumption, the greater the risk of this happening.

The body, however, has defense systems that are designed to help prevent this errant oxidation from causing any harm. But to be at their best, our defenses depend on a daily supply of *"antioxidant" nutrients,* which include vitamin C, the carotenoids, vitamin E, selenium, and zinc. These nutrients are found in fruits, vegetables, and grains.

Some Fats Are Essential

Although we need to limit the amount of fat we eat, it's important to understand that some fats, called essential fatty acids (EFAs), are essential to good health. Having these essential fatty acids in the diet can influence many of today's major maladies, including heart disease, high blood pressure, rheumatoid arthritis, intestinal ailments, psoriasis, and the complications from diabetes.

At present we know of at least two types of EFAs, the omega-3 and omega-6. The *omega-3 EFAs* come primarily from fish oils but can also be found in flaxseed (linseed) and to a lesser degree in walnut and canola oils. The *omega-6 EFAs* come primarily from vegetable seed oils, such as corn, soy, and safflower. We have learned that the body uses the EFAs to make powerful hormone-like compounds called prostaglandins (PGs). These PGs help determine how the body operates.

The typical American diet tends to be high in the omega-6 EFAs and too low in dietary omega-3s. This is an important point, because while both EFAs are essential, they have dramatically different health effects.

For example, a heart attack is caused when a blood clot blocks the flow of blood through an artery. The omega-6 PGs tend to encourage blood clotting, while those made from omega-3s inhibit the process. Experiments have shown that when more omega-3-containing fish are present in the diet, blood clots form at a slower rate and the incidence of heart attacks is significantly less.

Blood pressure is another topic of interest. It's beginning to look as if the PGs coming from the omega-3s can help moderate high blood pressure.

Both high blood pressure and blood clotting are involved in many long-term health complications seen with diabetes. Three recent reports make note of the potential benefits insulin-dependent diabetics may experience by eating more fish.

Having sufficient EFAs in the diet may also play a role in two disorders involving the immune system. In separate controlled studies—both preliminary—symptoms of rheumatoid arthritis and ulcerative colitis improved when volunteers were fed high levels of omega-3 EFAs in capsule form.

The omega-3 fats also have some potential as an anti-cancer agent. While the PGs produced from the omega-6 tend to increase tumor growth in experimental animals, those from the omega-3 from fish oil do not.

It's thought that diets high in fat represent a risk factor for cancer. Yet in those populations consuming a high-fat diet based on fish, the cancer levels are low. One study involving twenty-six countries discovered that the incidence of breast cancer decreased as fish consumption rose.

It is evident the omega-3 fats have a lot going for them. This underscores the need to include a dietary source, such as fish, in your diet.

But don't get the idea that one EFA is good and the other is bad. We need both of them. In fact, a study in the *Annals of Internal Medicine* told how a special omega-6 fatty acid extracted from the evening primrose and borage herbs, was effective in treating symptoms of rheumatoid arthritis for some individuals. Although most individuals can make this fatty acid, called gamma linolenic acid, in their bodies, it's believed that some are unable to make enough.

The problem with essential fats is that the typical American diet is way out of balance.

The omega-3 fats are available as a food supplement. Approach these with care, though, as the blood-clot-suppressing tendency of the omega-3s could leave one more susceptible to side effects ranging from nosebleeds to an increased risk of hemorrhagic stroke. It's best to rely on food such as nuts, seeds, vegetables, and fish as the source of healthful fats. Fish containing high levels of omega-3 EFAs include mackerel, sardines, salmon, tuna, herring, yellowtail, and trout.

How Much Fat Should You Eat?

For the average individual about thirty percent of the daily calories should come from fat. The number isn't as important as the overall makeup of the diet. If the diet is high in fruits, vegetables, legumes and whole grains, and there are not too many calories, the diet need not be restricted in terms of total fat. How, though, does "30 percent of calories" translate into actual grams of fat, the measure used on food labels? There are two quick methods that can be used.

The first, and perhaps simplest, method is to divide your ideal body weight by two. For example, the ideal body weight for a 5′ 4″ woman is about 130 pounds, and thus a daily fat allowance would be 65 grams (130 divided by 2). This method assumes a light to moderate activity level. While not very precise, the method does provide an answer with a minimum of math.

Another shorthand method relies on daily Calorie intake. Divide the number of Calories by 30 to get the maximum number of fat grams recommended. For example, someone on a 2,100-Calorie diet should have no more than 70 grams (2,100 divided by 30) of fat per day.

Calculating Percentage of Fat in Processed Foods

Although percentage of Calories from fat is not indicated on food labels, determining it is easy. The most accurate way is to divide the Calories from fat by the total Calories (both figures are listed under Amount Per Serving on the nutrition panel).

Another method uses grams of fat and Calories per serving. If there are no more than 3 grams of fat for every 100 Calories in a serving, then no more than 27 percent of the Calories are from fat—just below the recommended level. This formula works regardless of serving size.

Fat Content of Common Foods

1 cup broccoli	0 g
¹/₂ cup red kidney beans	0.4 g
1 cup rice	0.6 g
1 cup cooked pasta (no sauce)	1 g
1 slice sandwich bread	1 g
1 cup fruit-flavored yogurt	2 g
4 oz. fish (trout)	5 g
1 cup reduced-fat milk (2 percent)	5 g
1 large egg	5 g
1 cup marinara sauce	8 g
4 oz. roast chicken breast	9 g
1 cup tofu	9 g
1 tbsp. butter	12 g
1 oz. (20–30) almonds	14 g
2 tbsp. peanut butter	16 g
4 oz. hamburger	21 g
12 Oreo-type cookies	24 g

Keeping Some Perspective

As healthy eaters, our total fat intake should not be our only concern. We need to consider which fats we eat. When considering fats we need to rely more on monounsaturates and avoid partially hydrogenated fats whenever possible.

An understanding of the key players in the fat saga highlights how closely connected it is to an emphasis on fresh fruits, vegetables, grains, and nuts. With a balanced style of eating, you give the body the antioxidant nutrients it needs to protect itself. These healthful foods are the very ones that a high-fat diet tends to knock off the plate.

Spreading the Word on Hydrogenated Fats

While naturally occurring monounsaturated fats, such as olive, canola, and nut oils, are associated with a decreased risk of heart disease, stolidly perched at the other end of the spectrum we find partially hydrogenated fats. These semisolid processed fats have been solidifying their unhealthy reputation, primarily through evidence associating them with an increased risk of heart disease.

Food manufacturers make extensive use of partially hydrogenated oils—with good reason. At room temperature, oils (less saturated) are liquid, and fats (more saturated) are solid. The hydrogenation process can change an unsaturated oil into a solid block of saturated fat—but it usually doesn't go that far. The unsaturated vegetable oil, such as soy, corn, or canola, is "partially" hydrogenated into a semisolid fat. Through the hydrogenation process, a liquid vegetable oil is given a consistency suitable for wide variety of food products, including margarine and shortening, snack chips, cookies and crackers, pastries and puddings, and bread and breakfast cereals.

> Partial hydrogenation is not a totally benign process, no matter how useful it may be to food manufacturers.

During the hydrogenation process, an unusual breed of unsaturated fat called a trans fatty acid (TFA) is produced. Until recently, there wasn't widespread concern about TFAs. Because they are unsaturated fats, the majority of scientific opinion was that they posed little health risk. Now, however, TFAs are looking more and more like real troublemakers. Studies have found that TFAs tend to lower the level of high-density lipoproteins, or HDLs ("good" cholesterol), and raise the level of low-density lipoproteins, or LDLs ("bad" cholesterol)—both actions that contribute to an increased risk of heart disease.

In an article in the October 1997 *American Journal of Public Health,* Harvard researchers Dr. Walter Willett and Dr. Alberto Ascherio estimated that the partially hydrogenated fats found in margarine, shortening, and other processed foods are likely to account for an estimated 30,000 deaths a year from heart disease. Willett and Ascherio, both well-respected researchers, arrived at their number by analyzing the average U.S. intake of partially hydrogenated fats. They then factored in the estimated harm caused by these fats. Finally, they plugged in the yearly incidence of death from heart disease and came up with the likely toll contributed by the partially hydrogenated fat.

Another salvo against partially hydrogenated fats came from a year-long review by a specially commissioned Danish task force that was published in the journal *Clinical Science* in 1995. The task force concluded that the TFAs found in such foods as margarine contribute to heart disease at "the same or possibly to a higher extent than saturated fats." The report also found that trans fatty acids may "have a harmful effect on the growth of the fetus." The Danish Nutrition Council, which commissioned the task force, expressed hope that the findings would be "[looked upon as a] weighty document by the health authorities and the food industry."

Now, there's new evidence that what's good or bad for the heart may be having a similar effect on the risk of breast cancer. A 1995 study in the *Journal of the National Cancer Institute* uncovered important connections between breast cancer and a healthy diet. The strongest link was found between the intake of vegetables and fruits and a decreased risk of breast cancer. Similar to previous studies, no link was found between total fat consumption and the risk of the disease. A different picture emerged, however, when the fat components were looked at individually.

The scientist found a significant link between the consumption of olive oil and a decreased risk of the disease. No link was found between breast cancer and the consumption of butter, and none was found with seed oils. But when they examined the role of margarine—a partially hydrogenated product of these same seed oils—the scientists found that the level of intake was tied to an increased risk for the disease.

This is not the first time that the intake of partially hydrogenated fat has been linked to an increased risk of breast cancer. Population studies in Denmark and the Netherlands had previously found significant associations between the consumption of hydrogenated fat and the risk of breast cancer. And in a study presented at a national meeting for the American Society for Clinical Nutrition, scientists from the University of North Carolina reported on a link between trans fatty acids and the incidence of breast cancer. The study looked at 112 German women and relied on the TFA level in body fat to make its conclusions. A much larger multinational study is currently under way.

The possible link between partially hydrogenated fat and cancer may stem from the effect of the TFAs on two sets of opposing enzymes called the Phase 1 and Phase 2 enzymes, which are involved in the progress of human cancers. In a Japanese study, TFAs were found to stimulate the Phase 1 enzymes, the kind that tend to encourage the activity of cancer-causing substances.

Although these studies don't establish cause-and-effect, they provide yet another reason to be on the lookout for partially hydrogenated vegetable oils and zero them out of your diet whenever possible.

Implications for Industry and Agriculture

These findings are shaping up to be a major problem because partially hydrogenated fats are found throughout the food supply. As research continues to verify that partial hydrogenation adds an unnecessary health risk, the food industry could be facing consumer avoidance of the affected products.

Agriculture also has much at stake. Some of the country's largest cash crops, such as soybeans and corn, are used to form hydrogenated-oil products. If these findings have the expected impact on consumer demand, there will need to be a change in the amount of these vegetables grown for this purpose. At present, plant breeders are developing new lines of crops to contain types of fat that will lessen the dependency on hydrogenation. These developments, though, could be years away.

Avoiding TFAs

The best way to avoid TFAs is to control your intake of high-fat processed foods. Because most snack foods tend to be made with partially hydrogenated oils, these are the first ones to watch. Your use of shortening and spreadable vegetable fats should also be kept to a minimum. When using a spreadable fat, consider butter, or make your own "soft" spread by mixing butter with a liquid, monounsaturated oil such as canola, olive, or almond oil. If you are going to use margarine, choose a liquid or tub margarine—one that lists partially hydrogenated fat no higher than third on the ingredient statement. Ironically, canola-based margarines tend to have the highest TFA content.

A Trans Fatty Acid Sampler

Here's a list of some common foods made with partially hydrogenated fat, and the grams of TFAs they contain. As you read it, you can understand the difficulty in swallowing the previous estimates that the average TFA intake in this country was under 8 grams per day. Where do you think you stand?

Partially Hydrogenated Fat Content

1 tbsp. butter	0.5 g
1 tbsp. vegetable shortening	2.7 g
1 tbsp. margarine	3.5 g
12 soda crackers*	5.2 g
1 plain doughnut*	5.5 g
1 serving fried fish*	5.7 g
3½ oz. tortilla chips*	7.7 g
1 serving fried chicken*	7.8 g
4 oz. gourmet muffin*	8.2 g
1 large order french fries*	9.2 g
3½ oz. serving potato chips*	10.4 g
12 Oreo-type cookies	16.9 g
12 pecan sandies-type cookies	26.5 g

---

*When made with hydrogenated vegetable shortening.

The Fat Facts of Fried Foods

The frying oils in fast-food restaurants may have come originally from vegetables, but they retain few of the benefits of their origin. To meet the special demands of commercial deep-fat frying, these oils are changed through partial hydrogenation, a process by which liquid vegetable oil is modified to various consistencies for food products. And although fried foods never claimed to be health foods, this even further tarnishes their image.

Frying oil, similar to the hot air in an oven, is nothing more than a heat-transfer medium. The main difference between the oven and the deep-dryer is that cooking oil interacts with the food and lends a unique taste and texture.

Unlike heated air in an oven, though, cooking oil begins to break down as soon as it's used. When an oil breaks down, a mixture of by-products, including vitamin destroyers, stomach irritants, enzyme inhibitors, mutagens and lipid oxidation products, begin to form and hitch a ride with the fried-fat Calories of the food. The more unsaturated the oil, the faster the breakdown.

When we fry or sauté foods at home, a pure, unsaturated vegetable oil, such as peanut, corn, olive, or canola, can be taken straight from the bottle and discarded after use. As long as the oil isn't overheated, the breakdown is negligible.

But such vegetable oils don't have what it takes to withstand the rigors of commercial frying. In fast-food restaurants, for example, oils are kept at high temperatures and used continually throughout the day. The rate of breakdown increases as the oil is repeatedly used, and it accelerates if any food debris is allowed to remain in the hot oil. An unprocessed vegetable oil would rapidly deteriorate in this setting.

Saturated fats, by contrast, tend to be more stable, making it less likely that these nasty by-products will form. In addition, less fat is absorbed into the food during frying. That's why, for a long time, the main fats found in deep-fat fryers were beef tallow and saturated tropical oils such as coconut and palm oil. They should have left well enough alone.

In the early 1980's, under pressure from well-meaning consumer activists, fast food restaurants switched from their stable saturated frying fats to ones based on vegetable oils. The move was made to reduce the level of saturated fat in the American diet and, at the same time, banish another minor source of dietary cholesterol.

The use of vegetable oil lent a misguided aura of healthfulness to foods having only meager dietary assets at best, but the change was fraught with deception. Because of their impracticality, pure vegetable oils never made it into the fryer. It was as impractical then as it is now. In their place were oils that were partially hydrogenated to make them last longer.

> The trans fatty acids now swimming around in the restaurant deep-fat fryer are linked to major diseases such as heart disease and cancer. Too bad they don't just stay in the fryer.

French-fried foods made in partially hydrogenated oil contain eight times the TFAs that were present when beef tallow was predominantly used. Considering that the french fry is among the most popular items in the restaurant industry, the switch has likely had a significant impact on our health. Going back to the frying oils that were in use before partial hydrogenation invaded the deep-fat fryer is as good a place as any to start.

What's a Canola?

Canola is a type of vegetable oil which, by food standards, has come on the scene rather suddenly. What's unique about canola is that, unlike other vegetable oils, it didn't originate from a plant or seed of the same name. So what is a "canola"?

Canola stands for: *CAN*adian *O*il, *L*ow *A*cid. It's an oil derived from the seed of the rape plant, a member of the mustard family and a common crop in—you guessed it— Canada.

The oil of common varieties of the rape plant has a high concentration of erucic (ee-ROOS-ik) acid, a substance suspected of having a toxic effect in large amounts. Because of this, the oil was originally used mainly for industrial applications. But plant breeders were successful in developing a variety of rapeseed in which the erucic acid was virtually eliminated. Taking its place was a high concentration of oleic acid, the monounsaturated fat found in olive and other nut oils.

Given the growing body of research on the health advantages of using monounsaturated fats in a low-fat diet, the new hybrid rapeseed oil became a perfect product for foods. But who would buy a product named, "rape oil or rapeseed oil"? And the name "low-erucic-acid rapeseed oil" was thought to be too much of a mouthful. This set the stage for a new name, "canola."

In 1985, the oil received a GRAS (Generally Regarded As Safe) status from the U.S. Food and Drug Administration. In 1988, the name canola, by which it was known in Canada, was given approval for use in this country. Presto! A new word was added to the food vocabulary.

3. Carbohydrates:

From the Simple to the Complex

Protein, and especially fats, are often preceded by the advisory to "avoid too much," but there's been little constraint placed on carbohydrates. This is ironic, for it wasn't too long ago that carbohydrates—especially sugar—were on the hot seat, saddled with the blame for such common ailments as obesity, heart disease, and hyperactivity in children. Recently, however, science has cleared carbohydrates of their alleged nutritional misdeeds. Let's take a closer look at carbohydrates to see what they do.

Carbohydrates are the most plentiful nutrient substances in nature. The word comes from the Latin *carbo,* for carbon, and *hydras,* which refers to the combining with water. As a group, carbohydrates constitute the body's most important source of energy. There are three basic types: simple carbohydrates, complex carbohydrates, and fiber.

The most important carbohydrate is *glucose,* also called blood sugar. Glucose is the body's basic fuel: It's the preferred fuel of the brain and nervous system, and the only fuel that the red blood cells can use. Indeed, there are entire body systems dedicated specifically to maintaining the level of glucose in the blood.

Glucose is referred to as a single sugar because it exists as individual, unattached units. Other common single sugars in our diet include fructose, also called fruit sugar, and galactose.

Simple carbohydrates can be single sugars or double

sugars, so named because they consist of two single sugars attached to one another. The most common of the double sugars are sucrose, or table sugar (glucose attached to fructose); lactose, or milk sugar (glucose attached to galactose); and maltose (glucose attached to another glucose), which is found in grains and malt beverages such as beer. The taste sensation of sweetness comes from the ability of these single and double sugars to stimulate the sweet taste receptors on the tongue.

Simple carbohydrates undergo little in the way of digestion. The single sugars are absorbed intact and the double sugars must first be split apart. Because glucose is the body's energy "currency," it is up to the liver to change both fructose and galactose into glucose.

Glucose also serves as the building block for the complex carbohydrates that are found in grains, legumes, and potatoes. These *complex carbohydrates,* or starches, consist of hundreds to thousands of glucose units connected to each other in straight-line or branched formations. They are too large to be absorbed through the wall of the digestive tract, so the body relies on its digestive enzymes to break the starch apart, piece by glucose piece. These enzymes are specialized in that the one that works on the straight-line links doesn't work on the branches.

Cellulose, such as that found in hay and wood pulp as well as in many vegetables, is also made from glucose. The big difference, though, between digesting a meal of mashed potatoes and one of mashed wood is that while our body can take apart the glucose units of potato starch, we lack the appropriate enzymes to separate the glucose units of cellulose. As a result, starch gets digested and absorbed, and the cellulose passes through the system. Because the body cannot digest cellulose, this complex carbohydrate is classified as a dietary fiber.

Fiber is an umbrella term referring to a group of complex carbohydrates that have no nutrient value because they, like cellulose, are not digested. Despite this fact, this group, which includes cellulose, pectin, and vegetable gums, has taken on increasing importance as a crucial component in a healthy diet. Fiber is discussed in detail in chapter 4.

As an energy source, carbohydrates have a very special quality. Normally, muscles require oxygen from the bloodstream when they work. This is why our breathing rate picks up during physical activity. Carbohydrates are different from fats, the body's main fuel, because they release their energy anaerobically (*an*=without; *aerobic*=requiring oxygen). There's a small amount of stored carbohydrate, called glycogen, in the muscles and liver, and the body relies on this fuel to meet special demands. It's this fuel and the anaerobic ability of carbohydrates that enables us to dash across a room and grab a falling child or sprint down the street to catch a bus. Carbohydrates provide a vital source of energy that keeps the muscles working until the lungs gear up to provide the needed oxygen.

Focus on the Complex

When thinking about the carbohydrates in your diet, it's important to focus on the complex rather than the simple sugars. Why, you might ask, if all carbohydrates end up as glucose? The answer is in the nutrient company the different carbohydrates keep. Except for fruits, foods high in simple sugars tend to also be high-Calorie and often high-fat processed foods where intense flavor or a sweet taste is the main offering. Complex carbohydrates, by contrast, are generally found in grains, vegetables, and legumes—whole foods with a wide array of valuable nutrients and fiber.

Carbohydrates' Role in Nature's Energy Cycle

In essence, carbohydrates deliver energy from the sun to satisfy the needs of the body. In the process called photosynthesis, plants use energy from the sun and produce glucose from carbon dioxide and water in their environment. The plants then use the glucose as a building block for their growth. When we eat plants for food, the cells in our bodies make use of the glucose as fuel. To use the energy in glucose, the body breaks the glucose back down to carbon dioxide and water. The energy in the glucose is then released and used by our body. The water is either exhaled in our breath or excreted as urine, and the carbon dioxide returns to the air—both again available to be used by plants.

How Much Should You Eat?

For the average individual, one-half to two-thirds of the Calories eaten every day should come from vegetable, fruit, and grain-based carbohydrates. For an individual on a 2,000-Calorie diet, this translates to 250 to 335 grams of carbohydrates per day (there are 4 Calories in each gram of carbohydrate). The "bulk" of your intake should be from complex carbohydrates.

The Glycemic Index: How Different Carbohydrates Affect the Body

The glycemic index is a way of rating foods according to how fast and how high they cause your blood glucose to rise. This index was developed for use by diabetics and others, such as hypoglycemics, who have problems regulating their blood sugar level.

Carbohydrate Content of Common Foods

	Complex	Simple	TOTAL
1 cup rice	59 g	0 g	59 g
1 medium potato	48 g	3 g	51 g
1 cup red kidney beans	40 g	0 g	40 g
1 cup cooked pasta (no sauce)	40 g	0 g	40 g
1 medium sweet potato	15 g	13 g	28 g
1 cup Cheerio's cereal	15 g	1 g	16 g
1 slice whole-wheat bread	12 g	1 g	13 g
1 cup Sugar Smacks cereal	12 g	21 g	33 g
1 medium banana	9 g	18 g	27 g
1 medium carrot	3 g	4 g	7 g
1 medium orange	3 g	12 g	15 g
12 oz. cola soft drink	0 g	38 g	38 g
1 tbsp. granulated sugar	0 g	12 g	12 g

When the blood sugar level rises above its normal range—usually a signal that we've just eaten—the pancreas releases insulin. Insulin is the hormone that keeps the blood sugar level from getting too high. When insulin is present, glucose is removed from the blood. A small amount might be used for energy, or turned into glycogen, but most will probably be turned into fat, the body's form of stored energy. The larger the amount of sugar that hits our system at one time, the greater the amount of insulin and the greater the amount of fat that will be formed. The conversion is a one-way street, and once made, the fat is shuttled through the bloodstream in lipoproteins, those special "fat" carriers that contain cholesterol. Although studies have failed to make a connection between sugar consumption and heart disease, a high-sugar diet would not be wise for those at high risk for heart disease.

Diabetes occurs when, for any of a number of reasons, there's insufficient insulin to do the job. As a result, diabetics have to monitor their sugar and carbohydrate consumption as their inability to control a rising blood sugar level can have disastrous consequences. There are different types of diabetes—some require insulin injections, while others can be controlled using diet and oral medications. Although excess sugar has not been shown to directly cause diabetes, sugar, insulin, and diabetes are closely connected. If diabetes runs in your family, it would be prudent for you to limit your sucrose intake.

To control their blood sugar level, diabetics have to take either shots or pills to help provide the insulin they need. Hypoglycemia, by contrast, is the tendency to overrelease insulin. This causes the blood glucose level to drop more rapidly than normal, resulting in a level that's below the normal range. Diabetics and hypoglycemics have to closely monitor their sugar consumption, keeping it to an absolute minimum.

Knowing about the glycemic index can be of particular help to these individuals because it indicates which carbohydrate (glucose-containing) foods have the most rapid effect on blood glucose. In the traditional index, glucose is assigned a score of 100 percent and other foods are compared to that.

The glycemic index can be useful for foods eaten on an empty stomach, but it has limited usefulness for mixed meals. This is because the glucose from carbohydrate-containing foods is not absorbed until after it leaves the stomach. Because the presence of fat and, to a lesser degree, protein will delay stomach emptying, when carbohydrate foods are a part of a meal that contains fat, their effect on blood glucose will be less dramatic. This helps explain why a sweet snack food, such as ice cream, can have a low glycemic index. If, however, it was a low-fat or fat-free ice cream, the glycemic index would be much higher. Another limiting factor is the size of the meal. Eating many small meals can spread glucose absorption throughout the day and blunt the effect of any one meal.

Glycemic Index

100 percent:	glucose
80–90 percent:	instant mashed potatoes, raw carrots, puffed rice, cornflakes, parsnips, honey
70–79 percent:	white and whole-wheat bread, white rice, mashed potatoes, corn chips
60–69 percent:	rye bread, bananas, shredded wheat, brown rice, raisins
50–59 percent:	spaghetti, peas, corn, potato chips, frozen peas, yams, potato chips
40–49 percent:	oranges, orange juice, whole-wheat spaghetti, oatmeal, sweet potatoes
30–39 percent:	apples, milk, most beans, chickpeas, ice cream, yogurt
20–29 percent:	lentils, kidney beans, granulated fructose
10–19 percent:	peanuts, soybeans

4. Fiber for Health

Dietary fiber is a type of carbohydrate that's found only in plant products, such as vegetables, nuts, fruits, and grains. Although it is a key component of a healthy diet, it is not tied to any one benefit. Nutrition research has associated a high-fiber diet with a lower risk of diabetes, diverticulitis, hemorrhoids, ulcerative colitis, certain forms of cancer, and coronary heart disease. Fiber is also commonly used as a remedy for constipation.

That's an imposing set of talents, and it's particularly impressive when you consider that fiber does not contribute any Calories, essential vitamins, or minerals to the body. In fact, it's not digested by the body at all! How can a substance we can't even digest be so healthful? The very fact that you can't digest it is what turns out to be its greatest asset.

How Fiber Works

If we think of food as nutrients linked together by padlocks, digestion is the process of opening the locks. It is only after the chain is broken into smaller pieces that the body can absorb and use the nutrients. Digestive enzymes are the keys that open the locks. Fiber is unique because the body lacks the right keys to open its locks. This means that instead of being absorbed, fiber becomes part of the bulk that passes through the entire digestive system and eventually is eliminated from the body.

The word *fiber* is really an umbrella term. As it travels through the body, what fiber does depends on how it's built. An important distinction is whether the fiber dissolves in water; so there are two types of dietary fiber: *insoluble* and *soluble,* and their health benefits differ.

The most familiar of the insoluble fibers is wheat bran, but this type is also in vegetables, fruits, and whole grains, such as corn, rye, barley, and brown rice. Insoluble fiber increases the bulk and weight of the stool as well as the rate at which food travels through your digestive system. This makes for potential benefits against cancer. Population studies routinely find that the incidence of colon cancer decreases as the intake of insoluble fiber goes up. That's because fiber can effectively dilute or even bind potential cancer-causing substances and quickly usher them out of the body. Insoluble fiber can also help lower the risk of heart disease because its ability to bind the bile acids causes more cholesterol to leave the body.

Soluble fiber is found in oat and rice bran, legumes (beans, lentils, and peas), fruits, and vegetables. Although these fibers dissolve in water, the body cannot absorb them because they're large carbohydrates and the body lacks the enzymes to break them apart. Soluble fiber can't match the ability of insoluble fiber to add bulk. It can, however, improve conditions connected with diabetes because it tends to slow the rate at which the body absorbs sugar. In addition, through a complex series of reactions, soluble fiber has a demonstrated ability to help lower blood cholesterol levels. You'll notice that fruits and vegetables contain both soluble and insoluble fiber. This is further testimony to the wisdom behind including them in the diet.

Fiber Against Disease

A couple of recent studies reveal the potential health benefits of a high-fiber diet. First, a 1996 study in the *Journal of the American Medical Association* reported on the relationship between vegetable, fruit, and cereal fiber and the risk of heart disease. The study followed 43,757 male health professionals, forty to seventy-five years of age, for a period of six years. The research found a strong relationship between an increased fiber intake and a lower incidence of heart disease.

The study was noteworthy in that it eliminated any possible interference from factors such as smoking, physical activity, level of dietary fat, alcohol, and vitamin E. The JAMA study found cereal fiber to be the most effective at decreasing the risk of heart disease. Independent of the fiber effect, those who consumed at least five servings of fruits and vegetables a day had a significantly lower risk than those having less than three servings a day. This last finding reflects the fact that there are other heart-healthy factors found in fruits and vegetables.

The other study, in the 1996 *Journal of the National Cancer Institute* found beneficial effects from wheat bran on the risk of colon cancer. That study looked at ninety-five men and women, fifty to seventy-five years of age. All had previously had polyps removed from their large intestine, or colon. Polyps are abnormal growths that develop from the tissue that lines the colon. Although most prove to be harmless, virtually every cancer of the colon or rectum had to begin as a polyp. At present, it is estimated that up to 50,000 Americans die from colon cancer every year.

The subjects were randomly assigned to groups that received either a high-fiber cereal (13.5 grams of fiber per box), or a low-fiber cereal (2 grams of fiber per box), with either a high-calcium supplement (250 milligrams calcium carbonate) or a placebo calcium supplement (0 milligrams calcium carbonate). The study was "blind" in that subjects did not know which treatment they were receiving. The subjects were examined at three and nine months and the level of bile acids from their intestines were checked. After nine months, those receiving the high-fiber cereal had significantly lower levels of bile acids.

What are "bile acids" and what do they have to do with colon cancer? Bile is one of the digestive juices in our intestines. It plays a key role in fat digestion, helping to break food fats into very small globules to aid in their digestion and absorption. The bile is manufactured by the liver from cholesterol and it's stored in the gall bladder until needed. As a fat-containing meal leaves the stomach, bile travels through the bile duct and mixes with the meal in the small intestine.

Although the details of the process are not clearly understood, studies have connected high concentrations of bile acids with the risk of colon cancer. One theory states that the high concentrations of bile acids can increase the growth of cells in the large intestine. Having rapidly growing cells in the large intestines is not a good idea because the cells could then be exposed to any cancer-causing chemicals that might be present in the waste products about to be eliminated from the body. If this theory holds, fiber's beneficial effects could be due to its ability to bind the bile acids, which effectively decreases the contact time they might have with the intestinal wall.

If these studies do one thing, it is to lend further credence to the wisdom behind opting for high-fiber alternatives in your food selections. And, of course, both make a strong case for starting off the day with a high-fiber cereal.

How Much Fiber Should You Eat?

At present, the American public consumes only about 12 to 15 grams of dietary fiber per day. I recommend doubling this to *at least* 25 to 30 grams. To illustrate how important this could be, the JAMA study found that by adding 10 grams of fiber per day, the average individual would reduce their risk of heart disease an impressive 20 percent.

Fiber Sources	
1 slice whole-wheat bread	2 g
1 cup raw spinach	2 g
1/2 cup all-bran cereal	13 g
1 medium carrot	2 g
1 cup Cheerios	1 g
1 oz. almonds	3 g
1 tbsp. oat bran	1 g
1/2 cup dried figs	9 g
1 cup white rice	1 g
1/2 cup dried apricots	5 g
1 cup brown rice	3 g
1 medium apple	3 g
1 medium potato with skin	5 g
1 banana	3 g
1 medium sweet potato	3 g
1 cup broccoli	4 g
1 cup red kidney beans	15 g
1 tbsp. peanut butter	1 g

Consider Dried Fruit

Dried fruit is a fabulous, often overlooked source of fiber. Figs and dates contain 9 grams of fiber per half-cup serving, prunes contain 7 grams per serving, and apricots and raisins contain 5 grams. By comparison, a slice of whole-wheat bread or a 1/2 cup of broccoli contain about 2 grams of dietary fiber.

Besides its fiber content, dried fruit is also an excellent source of B vitamins and minerals. The pick of the group is the fig. Prized since the time of the pyramids, figs are one of the richest nondairy sources of calcium. One serving of figs contains 144 milligrams of calcium, which on an ounce-by-ounce basis places them higher than milk. Figs are also a good source of iron, vitamin B_6, magnesium, and copper. Apricots are also a definite standout, because one serving provides 25 percent of the U.S. RDA for iron and enough beta-carotene to satisfy almost 75 percent of the RDA for vitamin A.

These high-fiber fruits make a delicious and nutritious snack at home, in a child's lunch box, or stashed in a drawer for a workday nibble. They're also good chopped up in cottage cheese or yogurt, or in cereals or pancake mixes, where they can eliminate the need for added sugar. By rotating among the different fruits, you lend flavor and variety to the morning routine while adding nutritional value to the meal.

Because these are high-fiber foods, it's best not to abruptly add any large quantities to your daily diet; the result could be an overstimulated digestive system and a case of diarrhea. Try starting with a small serving and work up to a comfortable level. Portion control may also be needed with children. My son, for example, loves apricots, figs, prunes, and raisins. Of late, he has grown particularly fond of dried cranberries and dried mangoes. He'd eat as much as I'd let him have.

Be wary, however, of fruit rolls and all those other types of fabricated fruit doodads aimed at youngsters. These pseudo-fruits use popular children's characters, such as Ghostbusters, Ninja Turtles, and Mario Brothers, as well as dinosaurs, clowns, and jet fighters. The apparent aim is to cajole parents into choosing the products as a convenient way to add fruit to their children's diet. Although these products boast being made with "real fruit," they're primarily a gummy fiberless sugar concoction that pales in comparison to the genuine article.

Fiber Supplements

For years, people have been taking fiber supplements to relieve periodic constipation. Supplement use became more common as information on fiber's other benefits became known, especially soluble fiber's cholesterol-lowering potential.

It's important to understand, however, that when you add concentrated fiber to the diet, there is a greater chance of side effects such as bloating, cramps, diarrhea, and gas. In addition, loading up on fiber can interfere with the absorption of nutrients. This is a particular problem with supplements such as psyllium, the soluble fiber found in Metamucil (a popular over-the-counter aid intended for the relief of constipation). Medications may also be affected, so touch base with your health professional before adding any fiber supplements to your diet.

To add fiber to your diet, it's best not to rely on supplements. It makes more health sense to gradually shift to a diet based on fresh foods, with plenty of fruits, vegetables, legumes, and whole grains.

5. Vitamins and Minerals:
From A to Zinc

It wasn't until 1860 that scientists discovered that germs could be responsible for disease. Following that development, scientific energy shifted toward finding the bugs behind every illness. This approach wasn't always successful. Some illnesses seemed to persist even though all known germs were under control. The idea that the answer might lie with what people were eating (or not eating) was not as popular a concept as the "germ theory." But as time went by, more and more scientists began to look to food for their answers.

The history of vitamin and mineral nutrition contains many colorful tales of discovery. Some began with an investigation of the power certain foods seemed to have over disease; others came from failed growth experiments, where all the nutrients thought to be essential were present in the diet.

Vitamins

The word *vitamin* was coined in 1912 by Dr. Casmir Funk, a Polish scientist who was searching for a cure for beriberi, a paralyzing disease that was common in regions where white rice was the main staple in the diet. Earlier work had zeroed in on rice polishings—the husk and bran that are removed when brown rice is made into white—as containing some factor that could combat beriberi. Funk eventually identified the key compound, called thiamin, and dubbed it a "vital amine." This was shortened to "vitamin," which continues to stand for the entire class of essential compounds.

Vitamins are a diverse group of chemicals, but they have a few things in common:

- Compared with other nutrients, vitamins are needed only in trace amounts. All the required daily vitamins could fit in $1/8$ teaspoon.
- Vitamins do not provide any dietary energy (Calories).
- All vitamins are "organic," because they're based on the element carbon.
- Vitamins perform specific metabolic functions in the cell—the basic unit of life.
- Vitamins cannot be synthesized by the body in quantities large enough to meet the body's needs.
- Their absence from the diet leads to a failure to thrive and the development of a deficiency disease.
- All vitamins can be found in food.

Not all animals require the same vitamins. For example, humans are among the few animal groups that cannot manufacture their own vitamin C (ascorbic acid). This means your dog or cat does not need a daily ration of ascorbic acid, but you do.

Water-Soluble Vitamins

Vitamins are divided into two main categories, based on whether they dissolve in water. If we take in more of these vitamins than the body needs, the excess tends to be eliminated through the urine. Here are the water-soluble vitamins, what they do in the body, and a list of good food sources:

Thiamine (vitamin B_1): Needed for carbohydrates to release energy; also required for normal functioning of the heart and the nervous system. *Sources:* pork, liver, meat, fish, poultry, eggs, whole grains, legumes, nuts, and potatoes.

Riboflavin (vitamin B_2): Required for metabolism and energy release from food; important for health of the skin, the lining of the digestive system, and the lungs. *Sources:* liver, milk (enriched) and milk products, meats, seafood, enriched grains, asparagus, broccoli, avocados, Brussels sprouts, eggs, and green leafy vegetables.

Niacin (vitamin B_3, nicotinic acid, and nicotinamide): Required for normal cell metabolism and energy release from carbohydrates; also plays a role in the synthesis of hormones and DNA. *Sources:* organ meats, poultry, seafood, nuts, green vegetables, and legumes.

Pantothenic acid (vitamin B_5): Needed for energy release from food and for the synthesis of adrenal hormones and other chemicals involved in the nervous system. *Sources:* organ meats, milk products, egg yolk, poultry, mushrooms, nuts, green vegetables, and whole grains.

Pyridoxine (vitamin B_6): A key vitamin in protein metabolism; also plays a role in fat and carbohydrate metabolism. *Sources:* blackstrap molasses, meat, organ meats, poultry, wheat germ, brewer's yeast, whole grains, fish, soybeans, bananas, avocados, green leafy vegetables.

Vitamin B_{12}: With folic acid, helps to form red blood cells; needed for healthy nervous tissue and manufacture of genetic material. *Sources:* meat, poultry, fish, shellfish, eggs, dairy products, vitamin B_{12}-fortified foods, and fermented soy products.

Ascorbic Acid (vitamin C): Needed for healthy gums, wound healing, and to make collagen (the "cement" that holds body cells together). Also serves as an antioxidant, and plays a role in the immune system, protein metabolism, and other body systems. *Sources:* citrus fruits, peppers, melons, berries, Brussels sprouts, green vegetables, tomatoes, and potatoes.

Folic Acid: With vitamin B_{12}, helps make red blood cells; important for the manufacture of genetic material. *Sources:* green leafy vegetables, organ meats, legumes, orange juice, beets, avocados, and broccoli.

Biotin: Needed for metabolism and synthesis of fats, amino acids, and carbohydrates. *Sources:* organ meats, oatmeal, egg yolk, milk, soybeans, peanuts, whole grains, fruits, and vegetables.

The missing numbers in the B series reflect the inexactness of science. Over the years there were many "discoveries" of water-soluble vitamins that later turned out to be false. Some had already been assigned a number in the B series, so when they were finally rejected, the number was discarded as well.

Fat-Soluble Vitamins

There are four fat-soluble vitamins: A, D, E, and K. Beta-carotene, which can be transformed by the body into vitamin A, is not considered a vitamin in its own right. Unlike water-soluble vitamins, fat-soluble vitamins are not excreted through the urine; they remain in body tissues until they are either used up or broken down. Here is a description of their functions in the body, along with some good food sources:

Vitamin A (retinol or beta-carotene): Needed for proper vision and skin health; has antioxidant abilities and may protect against infection and certain cancers. *Sources:* liver and fish liver oils, vitamin A-fortified foods, egg yolk; beta-carotene found in carrots, green leafy vegetables, sweet potatoes, squash, apricots, and cantaloupes.

Vitamin D: Needed for healthy bones and teeth—necessary for the absorption of dietary calcium. *Sources:* fortified dairy products, fish, fish oils, egg yolk; also manufactured by body when directly exposed to sunlight.

Vitamin E (tocopherol): As an antioxidant, vitamin E protects fats and cell membranes from free-radical destruction; also helps form red blood cells. *Sources:* wheat germ, nuts and seeds, whole grains, vegetable oils, and green leafy vegetables.

Vitamin K: Required for normal blood clotting. *Sources:* turnip greens and other leafy vegetables, cruciferous vegetables, whole grains, and green tea.

When present in greater-than-required quantities, excess water-soluble vitamins are extracted by the kidneys and excreted in the urine. As a result, there is little danger from a long-term build-up of these compounds. With fat-soluble vitamins A and D, however, the body stores the excess in areas such as the liver or the fat tissue. If excessive amounts are continually taken, there's an increased risk of buildup to a toxic level.

Minerals

A mineral is loosely defined as anything in nature that is not animal or vegetable. For nutrition purposes, though, minerals are defined as follows:

- Minerals are inorganic chemical elements, in that they do not contain the element carbon.
- Minerals don't contribute any Calories.
- Relative to protein, fats, and carbohydrates, minerals are needed only in trace amounts.

- Minerals are required for use in specific structures or metabolic functions.
- Minerals are neither synthesized nor changed by the body.
- Their absence from the diet leads to a failure to thrive and the development of a deficiency disease.
- All essential minerals can be found in foods.

Minerals We Need

Of the fifteen required minerals, six are needed in relatively large amounts (hundreds of milligrams). These include calcium, phosphorous, magnesium, potassium, chloride, and sodium. The remaining nine are equally essential, but are needed in milligram or microgram amounts: iron, zinc, iodine, manganese, selenium, copper, fluoride, chromium, and molybdenum. Here is a list of the minerals, their functions in the body, and good food sources:

Calcium: Needed primarily for bones (99 percent of body calcium is in the bones) and teeth, but also for muscle contraction, normal heart rhythm, blood clotting, enzyme production, and nerve transmission. *Sources:* milk and milk products, green leafy vegetables, sardines and other small fish with edible bones, oysters, almonds, broccoli, dried figs and apricots, navy beans, tofu, almonds, brazil nuts, and blackstrap molasses.

Chloride: Forms digestive acid (hydrochloric acid—HCL) in the stomach; also one of the key elements in fluid and acid/base balance in the cells of the body. *Sources:* salt (sodium chloride), meat, fish, and poultry.

Chromium: Functions as part of glucose-tolerance factor, a substance that works with insulin to regulate blood-sugar level. *Sources:* whole grains, peanuts, organ meats, legumes, molasses, cheeses, and brewer's yeast.

Copper: Helps in the formation of red blood cells; essential for normal hair and skin; needed for antioxidant enzyme production and normal respiration. *Sources:* organ meats, shellfish, meats, legumes, nuts, raisins, and mushrooms.

Fluoride: Encourages hardness of bones of teeth and helps prevent tooth decay. *Sources:* fluoridated water, fish, and tea.

Iodine: Needed for normal activity of thyroid gland and essential for normal cell activities. *Sources:* seafood, sea vegetables, iodized salt, and foods grown on iodine-rich soil.

Iron: Needed for two oxygen-carrying compounds—hemoglobin in red blood cells, and myoglobin in muscle cells; also involved in the immune system. *Sources:* red meats, liver, egg yolk, poultry, fish, eggs, iron-fortified cereals, breads, rice, nuts, seeds, legumes, dried fruits, and some dark green leafy vegetables.

Magnesium: Needed for normal bones (half of body's magnesium is in the bones), and required for normal nerve transmission, muscle relaxation, and normal heart rhythm. *Sources:* nuts, bananas, legumes, whole grains, avocados, dark leafy greens, milk, and oysters.

Manganese: Helps in the formation of bones and connective tissue, and needed for normal metabolism, reproduction, and digestion. *Sources:* whole grains, tea, raisins, nuts, legumes, and leafy vegetables.

Molybdenum: Needed for key metabolic enzymes, helps form compounds required for iron utilization, and required for normal growth and development. *Sources:* whole grains, legumes, milk, and dark green vegetables (depends on soil content).

Phosphorous: Primarily found in bones and teeth, but widely distributed throughout body for general metabolism. Plays a role in energy transfer and is a part of the body's genetic material. *Sources:* meat, poultry, eggs, legumes, fish, whole grains, and nuts.

Potassium: Works with sodium to help regulate the

body's fluid balance; also needed for muscle contraction and normal heart rhythm. *Sources:* most fruits, legumes, vegetables, meats, and fish.

Selenium: Needed to create a key antioxidant enzyme that acts as a free-radical scavenger designed to protect against cell damage. *Sources:* seafood, whole grains and vegetables grown in selenium-rich soil, and organ meats.

Sodium: Works with potassium to help maintain fluid balance; also involved in the regulation of blood pressure. *Sources:* salt, seasoning salts, smoked and other cured foods, and most processed foods.

Zinc: Plays a role in many enzymes, including those involved in detoxification, sex-hormone production, and wound healing; also involved in taste and smell. *Sources:* shellfish, seafood, liver, meat, nuts, legumes, milk and milk products, eggs, whole grains, corn, and wheat germ.

It's dangerous to take too much of the minerals, especially where the trace elements are concerned. For example, there is a narrow margin of safety between the RDA for iron (18 milligrams for women) and the minimum adult toxic dose of 100 milligrams. Another reason to use caution is that minerals often work in conjunction with each other; taking an excess of a single mineral can throw off the body's delicate balance.

Do You Need a Supplement?

Since the days when potions were marketed by sideshow con artists, people have always been attracted to pills and powders that promise an extra boost. Given this, it's not surprising that many Americans look to supplements as a form of nutrition insurance. But do we need such insurance, or are the only beneficiaries the companies that sell the pills?

The supplement question is an important one because it goes to the heart of what nutrition and good eating are all about. The short answer is that it's unrealistic to think that supplements can capture all the goodness that healthful foods have to offer. This being said, however, the argument for taking supplementary antioxidants can be quite convincing. Let me explain.

The nutritional adequacy of the American diet has been a topic of debate since the first measurements of food consumption. The recommended dietary allowance (RDA) is defined as the level of intake that will satisfy the nutrient needs of practically all healthy persons. Most Americans, however, do not meet all the RDAs for vitamins and minerals on a daily basis. This in itself is not that serious a problem. The RDAs are not rigid requirements that must be met every day, but rather goals to be met as an average over time. There's little danger from missing a nutrient on a particular day so long as your intake over a five-to-ten-day period is at or near the RDA level.

> But what if we consistently fail to eat properly? Although we may never experience a full-blown deficiency disease, our chronically deficient diet is likely to have some negative effect on our health. If this is the case, isn't getting nutrients from a pill better than not getting them at all?

Yes, would seem to be a reasonable answer, but you won't find the surgeon general echoing this sentiment. Our conservative health establishment maintains a consistently thumbs-down attitude about vitamin and mineral supplements. Most consider the idea of supplements unscientific, potentially dangerous, and a waste of money. The use of a supplement might be justified for a small number of groups, such as people on very low-Calorie diets, those unable to absorb nutrients from their food, women with heavy menstrual bleeding, and women who are pregnant or lactating. But there has never been a category for people who simply do not eat well.

In recent years, however, food supplements have moved beyond their fill-in-the-gaps image. Evidence is mounting that extra amounts of some nutrients can be effective against common ailments and several age-related illnesses. For example, there's growing evidence that antioxidant vitamins, such as vitamins E and C, and the carotenoids are beneficial against heart disease, certain cancers, rheumatoid arthritis, and cataracts. Supplementary levels of the mineral calcium, besides slowing the onset of osteoporosis, has shown some ability to lower high blood pressure and prevent colon cancer. Niacin has been used alone and in combination with other medications against elevated blood cholesterol, fiber against colon cancer, and omega-3 fats (fish oils) against heart disease. Despite these scientific findings, there's no official acknowledgment that supplements have any value.

What could be behind this antipill stance? One possible answer is that by giving the nod to supplements, people might take the endorsement out of context. While a daily supplement can raise the intake of nutrients to recommended levels or beyond, an over-dependence on pills could change the way we think about food. It would be tragic if a "junk food plus supplements" diet began to look as good as one based on fresh, whole foods, because it doesn't even come close.

The healthfulness of eating fresh fruits, vegetables, and grains was verified through epidemiology, the science that investigates the connection between what people are eating or doing and their state of health.

The fact that good eating leads to good health is not news. What's relatively new is the technical ability to tweak out the identity of the compounds that make health-promoting foods work. To date, attention has focused primarily on a few minerals, dietary fiber, and antioxidant compounds such as vitamins E and C, and the carotenes. This is not because these are the only players, or because they are the most important; they simply were ones that scientists started working on first. Studies continue to appear touting the health benefits of other fruit and vegetable antioxidant compounds, such as the flavonoids (fruits and vegetables), isoflavones (soy), and polyphenols (wine and tea).

If you rely only on supplements, you will only get those nutrients that have been studied to the point that they have tickled the fancy of supplement makers enough to include them in their mix. Supplements cannot give you the full spectrum of what your body needs. Good food is the most reliable way to go.

This being said, however, the idea of supplements does have a lot going for it. In the case of vitamin E, for example, the average consumer would be hard-pressed to get enough in the diet (100 International Units) to come up to the level studies have found would be needed to achieve a significant reduction (40 percent) in the risk of heart disease. Similar arguments can also be made for vitamin C and the carotenes.

Research evidence seems to proclaim that those interested in good health had better have these nutrients in their diets on a regular basis. And, frankly, if you're not going to get them from the foods you eat, it's better to get them from a pill than not at all. To repeat, however, you will only be getting the benefits of these specific nutrients. They won't make a junk-food diet less junky, and it certainly doesn't come close to a diet based on fresh, whole foods.

Incidentally, most of us take vitamin and mineral supplements without even knowing it. Through fortification and enrichment, vitamins and minerals are added to processed foods. Breakfast cereals are a good example. The vitamins and minerals flaunted in ads don't come from the grain—they're added to the cereal formula before the final product is made. Cereals are not alone. Vitamin D is added to milk, fruit juices contain added vitamin C, and rice and most flours are enriched with thiamin, niacin, iron, and riboflavin.

Any vitamin or mineral listed on an ingredient statement is an indication that the nutrient was purposefully added to the product. The reason? Often it's to replace nutrients that were lost during processing. Sometimes, however, critical nutrients are added to commonly consumed food staples to reduce the danger of widespread deficiencies.

The bottom line is this: If you're interested in improving your eating habits, the first step is rarely found in a bottle of supplements. But so long as it's clearly understood that a vitamin/mineral pill cannot transform a poor diet into a healthy one, the decision to use a supplement can be an entirely reasonable one.

Natural or Synthetic?

The body cannot tell the difference between a natural vitamin and one that is synthetically made. Anyone that tells you different is not speaking from any science that I am aware of. One motivator to buy natural is to play on the disdain many have for the concept of "synthetic."

If there are benefits to natural over synthetic, they lie not in the vitamin but in *vitamin preparation* . . . the rest of the pill (or capsule), if you will.

Take beta-carotene: A pill of synthetic beta-carotene will *only* contain beta-carotene, while one from natural sources will likely contain other carotenes—even if it is not stated on the label.

Other touted aspects, such as of better absorbability, greater bioavailability, better for you, etc., are all theoretical, but they are possible. The proof, however must be established by the manufacturer using science, not marketing language such as "you can't put a price on health."

As to whether the promise of these qualities makes it worth the additional price—that's a question only you and your economic situation can answer. If the supplements were your only source of nutrients, I would say the natural sources would be better. But since you eat and probably are getting the "other" factors in the foods you eat, the natural supplement becomes less necessary from a nutritional perspective.

One final point is the quality of the formula. Synthetic formulas are often limited in their range of nutrients and in the potencies they offer. You can often be "forced" into buying more expensive supplements to get the formula you seek.

Planning Your Supplement Strategy

If you are constantly concerned with the adequacy of your diet, taking a supplement for nutrition insurance is not necessarily a bad policy. Before shopping for a supplement, however, it helps to know what you're looking for. Otherwise you risk being cut adrift in a sea of inflated claims and misinformation. Reading about the nutrients your body needs can help you better understand which, if any, you might be missing. In addition, you will learn about those nutrients that you might want to take at higher-than-required levels. With more information you may decide that a simple strategy, such as five servings a day of fruits and vegetables, is all that's needed to boost the nutrients in your diet.

If you feel that supplements would be of value, a basic multi-vitamin/mineral pill is a good place to start. Look for pills that contain 100 to 300 percent of the recommended dietary allowances. As freshness can affect vitamin potency, opt for brands that include expiration dates. (Note: A quick and convenient test to see if you're getting the nutrients out of your supplement is to put the pill in a half glass of warm vinegar. The pill should break apart within forty-five minutes.)

Be especially alert to exorbitant health claims made by those selling health products through multilevel marketing. For those unaware of this approach, it involves not only selling products, but trying selling you on the idea of selling the same products to others. If you agree, you become a part of that salesperson's organization and they benefit from all your activities. You, in turn, profit by your sales as well as the sales of anyone you might convince to sell products for you. The problem with this approach is that it mixes monetary incentives with promises for health benefits. In this setting, the substantiation for health claims is often given short shrift.

Finally, when you visit your physician, always be upfront about your use of supplements. This is necessary because some nutrient supplements can interfere with prescription medication, especially those with higher-than-RDA levels.

Folic Acid

Folic acid plays a key role in helping prevent anemia and certain types of birth defects. New research evidence has now found that this B vitamin can also play a role in decreasing the risk of heart disease. What's encouraging about folic acid's laudatory talents is that they don't rely on megadose amounts. You can get all the folic acid you need from a healthy diet. But, unfortunately, surveys indicate that folic acid-containing foods are apparently in dangerously short supply on the average U.S. plate. The best food sources for folic acid, also called folate, include dark green leafy vegetables, citrus fruits such as oranges, tomatoes, strawberries, beans, liver, peanuts, and folic acid-fortified cereals.

What's so special about folic acid? The body is in a constant state of flux, with cells being replaced on a regular basis. The raw materials for this cellular "turnover" comes, in part, from the body's own recycling system and partially from newly received materials. Folic acid is a key ingredient in a type of construction shuttle service that moves the body's single carbon "bricks" from one compound to another. Folic acid also plays a role in the synthesis of DNA and RNA, the genetic material involved in cell division and reproduction.

As you would imagine, when the construction of new cells and tissues goes awry, or is forced to slow down, there can be serious repercussions.

When folic is in short supply, one of the first places problems occur is in the blood. In cellular terms, the life span of the doughnut-shaped red blood cell is relatively short, each cell being replaced every 120 days. Because of this short life span, they are among the first cells in the body to suffer from a folic acid deficiency. Without folic, red blood cells are not made in sufficient numbers and a type of anemia results.

Giving a folic acid supplement or adding folic acid-rich foods can bring about a dramatic recovery in those suffering from a folate-deficiency anemia.

The outlook, however, isn't as promising if there's a folic acid deficiency during pregnancy. Following conception, the developing fetus begins to lay down the groundwork for many bodily systems. One of the first to develop is the nervous system, and folic acid plays a key role. The catch, though, is that folic acid must be present during the first few weeks after conception—a time at which most women are unaware they're even pregnant. If there's insufficient folic acid during this crucial period, mistakes can be made in the formation of the nervous system. Unfortunately, no amount of folic acid can make up for these structural abnormalities once that period has passed.

Spina bifida is a type of birth defect in which one or more of the vertebra of the spinal column fail to develop properly. It affects approximately one out of every 1,000 babies born. It is estimated that as much as 75 percent of all cases of spina bifida are attributable to a folic acid deficiency during those first few weeks of pregnancy. This makes it especially important for all women to have adequate folic acid in their diets *before* the pregnancy even begins. The problem is that less than half of all pregnancies are planned—this especially being true for young women.

> The U.S. Public Health Service recommends that all women of childbearing age who are capable of becoming pregnant should make sure they consume at least 400 micrograms of folic acid per day.

Now there's a new chapter on folic acid that involves its potential role in the prevention of heart disease.

Scientists have discovered that if the body doesn't have enough folic acid, a chemical called homocystine begins to accumulate. A number of studies have indicated that as the levels of homocystine rise, so too does the risk of heart disease.

A study in the *New England Journal of Medicine* looked

at 1,041 elderly men and women. The scientists at the USDA's Human Nutrition Research Center on Aging at Tufts University found that those with the highest levels of homocysteine in their bloodstream were twice as likely to have significant narrowing of the arteries in the neck— amounting to as much as a 25 percent loss of the inner diameter. Such a decrease in blood flow would be a serious harbinger to heart disease and stroke.

Once again, this is not the taking of *extra* folic acid, it's just giving the body what it needs. And, we don't seem to be doing a good job. The second National Health and Nutrition Education Survey (NHANES II) of food consumption found the average folic acid intake to be 200 micrograms per day—half the Public Health Service guideline. Now, whenever you talk of averages, it means there are those that have more and those who have less. Considering the serious implications of a chronic folic acid deficiency, something needs to be done to bring us all up to a safe level.

To help reduce all these serious, yet avoidable health risks, the Food and Drug Administration mandated the folic acid fortification of staple foods such as cereals, breads, and pastas, which began on January 1, 1998. A study in the *American Journal of Public Health* affirmed how grain fortification could prevent hundreds of birth defects every year.

Iron: The Mineral with Mettle

The body uses iron to make hemoglobin, an oxygen-carrying compound in the blood, as well as myoglobin, a compound that handles oxygen in the muscles. When there's not enough iron, the levels of hemoglobin and myoglobin decrease and with them goes the body's ability to produce energy. Anemia (*an*=without, *emia*=blood) is the most widespread deficiency disease in the world. It is marked by fatigue, headaches, dizziness, and a general "run down" feeling—symptoms often mistaken as normal side effects of a stressful lifestyle. The most common anemia type is an iron-deficiency that can be caused by a lack of iron in the diet, inefficient absorption of iron in the diet, or a loss of blood.

We see iron-deficiency anemia most often in groups where there's an increased iron need: children up to four years of age, teens during periods of rapid growth, women throughout the menstrual years and especially during pregnancy and lactation, frequent blood donors, endurance athletes, and anyone experiencing a significant loss of blood. Anemia can also result in people with disorders of the digestive system that affect the body's ability to absorb nutrients.

Iron in food comes in two groups: *Heme* iron, the type absorbed most efficiently, is present in red meats, poultry, fish, and eggs; *nonheme* iron sources include cereals and breads made with iron-enriched grains, nuts, seeds, legumes, dried fruits, and some dark green leafy vegetables. The U.S. RDA is 18 milligrams per day.

Iron Sources

1/2 cup dried apricots	8 mg
3 oz. cooked liver	6 mg
1 cup cooked spinach	5 mg
1 cup Cheerios cereal	4 mg
1/4 lb. lean ground beef	3 mg
1/2 cup red kidney beans	3 mg
1 tbsp. blackstrap molasses	3 mg
1/2 cup raisins	2 mg
1 oz. almonds	1 mg
1/2 cup raw oysters	8 mg

From this list, it's clear that iron is present in a variety of foods. Why, then, the continued prevalence of iron-deficiency anemia? One reason is that only a small percentage of dietary iron gets absorbed. In addition, there are naturally occurring chemicals in several foods, such as tea, coffee, whole grains, and some vegetables, that make iron unavailable to the body.

If you're among those with low iron or anemia, the logical first step is to include more iron-rich foods; the more meals containing iron, the better. Try having iron-rich meals along with high-acid fruits, such as oranges, or fruit juices high in vitamin C, because they enhance iron absorption.

There's some preliminary evidence that dietary calcium might inhibit the body's ability to absorb iron. So to play it safe, try to have at least one "iron" meal without coffee, tea, or calcium-containing foods or beverages, such as milk, cheese, and other dairy products. Those who are low in iron and are also taking calcium supplements should refrain from taking the calcium along with iron-containing foods.

During pregnancy and lactation, there's special emphasis on eating a healthy diet. Many women also take prenatal supplements with their meals as a form of nutrition "insurance." There's a loophole in the policy, though, because most supplements combine calcium and iron in the same pill. If iron is of special concern to you and your supplement contains both minerals, discuss with your physician the possibility of taking a separate iron supplement between meals or at bedtime.

Periodic use of cast-iron pans is an excellent way to add iron to the diet. When acid foods, such as spaghetti sauce, are prepared in cast iron, a small amount of iron dissolves into the food. The actual amount of iron drawn into food depends on the condition of the cookware; a cast-iron pan that's frequently seasoned with oil tends to give off less iron, although some iron will be released.

Can You Overload on Iron?

Yes, but it's not easy for the average individual. The body happens to be quite good at regulating its iron level. The protein needed for iron absorption is not available when the body's iron stores are full. There is, however, a genetic iron-storage disease called hemochromatosis. To have this condition you have to receive the gene from both your parents. In the United States, about one in ten has a single gene for this condition, and one in twenty-five has both genes. The condition is characterized by an inability to rid the body of excess iron. It is manageable through strict dietary control of iron-containing foods and periodic phlebotomy (blood donation). With the exception of individuals with hemochromatosis, it's highly unlikely that anyone could eat enough iron-containing foods to cause a toxic overdose. You could overdose on iron supplements, however, but only if you routinely ingested in excess of 100 milligrams of iron per day. It also might be possible if your daily diet included a hefty serving of high-acid foods, such as tomatoes, prepared in cast-iron cookware.

There's been speculation that too much iron could lead to heart attacks, but such a connection does not appear to be solid. We're familiar with the tendency of iron to rust, which results from its ability to react with oxygen. Although bodies don't get rusty per se, free iron could grab onto oxygen, then force it on nearby substances, such as fats or cholesterol. (It is these oxidized fats and cholesterol that are thought to be the real villains in heart disease.) But iron is rarely on its own in the body. Rather, it is tied up in such compounds as hemoglobin, the substance that makes red blood cells "red" and carries oxygen from the lungs directly to the cells. In addition, a well-nourished body should have a daily supply of antioxidant nutrients: vitamins C, E, and A and the carotenes. It's the responsibility of these nutrients to prevent the type of errant oxidation of which iron is being accused.

Selenium: From Checkered Past to Health Superstar

Selenium is a good example of a nutrient with a checkered past. Branded for decades as a dangerous toxin, selenium was later reclassified as an essential nutrient in the diet. There is new evidence that suggests selenium might be helpful against some of the most vexing diseases of our time: cancer and AIDS.

The selenium story can be traced to the middle of the nineteenth century and a mysterious condition called the blind staggers. It was known that cattle grazing in certain areas of the western United States would mysteriously go blind and develop an unsteady gait before they eventually died. In the 1930s, this puzzling illness was finally traced to unusually high levels of selenium in the soil and plants of the animals' grazing area.

It wasn't until 1957 that scientists confirmed that the body required selenium in small amounts. A landmark study described how selenium worked together with vitamin E to prevent damage to our cells.

We now know that selenium works as an antioxidant, the class of nutrients that helps protect the body against cell-damaging compounds called free radicals. Scientists believe that free-radical damage is involved in heart disease, cancer, and a host of other ailments, as well as in the aging process.

The body uses selenium to make a key protective enzyme called glutathione peroxidase. While other antioxidants (such as vitamins C and E, and beta-carotene) can help stop free radicals from forming, this selenium enzyme has the unique ability to stifle the free radicals once they've formed. It is also thought that selenium might have an ability to help stop the progression of tumors already in the body.

Over the years, selenium hasn't received the same attention as other essential nutrients, and I think that is unfortunate. Perhaps the reason is that selenium is only needed in minute amounts. The RDA for selenium was first established in 1989, and it is now set at 55 micrograms per day for adult women and 70 micrograms per day for men. (One microgram is one millionth of a gram!)

Low blood selenium levels are associated with an increased risk for cancer, heart disease, birth defects, and fibrocystic breast disease. The key is to take enough but not too much. An intake range of 50 to 200 micrograms a day is sufficient.

Selenium versus AIDS

In 1983, based primarily on evidence that selenium was effective against other viruses, Dr. Gerhard Schrauzer, now at the University of California at San Diego, suggested that selenium might be helpful in the fight against AIDS. The idea, however, didn't gather many supporters. As time passed, studies continued to report low blood selenium levels in AIDS patients. Recently new studies have focused interest on selenium as a potentially useful tool in the fight against AIDS.

One study published in the *Journal of Biological Chemistry* described a direct relationship between infection with the AIDS virus and a decreased activity of the selenium enzyme. Such a development is consistent with the type of free-radical destruction associated with the virus.

A second study, in the *Journal of Medicinal Chemistry,* speculated about how selenium might play a role in slowing down the uncontrolled growth of the AIDS virus. According to the theory suggested in the study, cells being infected with the AIDS virus would attempt to use selenium to help check the virus's growth. But the virus may be acting as a selenium "magnet," snatching the selenium for its own use. As the virus grabs the selenium, the paper theorizes, the cell becomes selenium-deficient, and in this state it's unable to stop the virus from proceeding along its destructive path.

Finally, a review paper by Dr. Schrauzer in *Chemico-Biological Interactions* gives evidence why selenium supplements may play an integral role in maintenance therapy for patients infected with the AIDS virus. He also suggests that adequate selenium may help reduce the risk of the AIDS virus being able to cross the placenta during pregnancy.

Selenium versus Cancer

(Additional discussion concerning diet and cancer can be found in Chapter 12.)

Recent research has found encouraging new evidence on the potential role for selenium in the fight against cancer. Previous studies have connected selenium with a lower risk of cancer. Then, a team of scientists led by Larry C. Clark, Ph.D., from the University of Arizona, designed a study to see if selenium supplements might be protective against skin cancer. As revealed in the *Journal of the American Medical Association,* the research did not find any protective effect against skin cancer, but those taking the selenium supplements had a significantly lower incidence of many other cancers and a lower cancer mortality in general.

The study followed a total of 1,312 patients who were considered to be at high risk for skin cancer because each had a history of one of two types of cancer; basal cell carcinoma or squamous cell carcinoma. If treated early, these types of skin cancers can usually be cured. Those having had malignant melanoma, a more life-threatening type of skin cancer, were not included in the study.

The initial objective of the study was to find out whether taking a supplement of the mineral selenium might be effective in preventing a recurrence of skin cancer. Using a double-blind, placebo-controlled design, half of the patients took a daily supplement that contained 200 micrograms of selenium supplied as 0.5 grams of high-selenium yeast (there are 1,000 micrograms in 1 gram). This is an organic source of selenium that is similar to that found in foods. The other half took a placebo. The patients took their pills for about 4.5 years and were monitored for an additional 6.4 years. Midway through the study it was decided to expand the objective of the study and collect data on other cancers in addition to skin cancer.

Although the results indicated that the selenium supplement didn't help protect against skin cancer, it had some rather impressive effects on cancers in general. When compared with those taking the placebo, the selenium group had a 37 percent reduction in the overall incidence of cancer and a 50 percent reduction in cancer mortality.

> Of the 200 new cases of cancer in the total patient population, the group taking the selenium supplement had 63 percent fewer prostate cancers, 58 percent fewer colorectal cancers, and 46 percent fewer lung cancers than the group taking the placebo.

Should You Take a Supplement?

Does this collection of research mean we should consider taking selenium supplements? At this point the scientists involved in the study are urging caution. It's not clear what it is about selenium that might be responsible for the protective effect experienced by the group taking the supplements. There may be some individuals who could use more selenium in their diets, but an overdose could do more damage than it could hope to prevent. In my opinion, however, the evidence attests to the importance of getting adequate selenium.

Food sources for selenium include Brazil nuts, seafood such as tuna, clams, oysters, swordfish, and lobster, organ meats, and grains such as oats and wheat. The selenium present in our foods, however, depends to a great degree on the selenium content of the soils or water in which they're grown. Selenium tends to be highest in soils west of the Mississippi River and east of the Rocky Mountains. Low selenium areas of the United States include the Northeast, the Pacific Northwest, and the southeastern coastal plains.

Selenium deficiencies tend to be uncommon in this country because we generally eat foods from many geographical areas. One study found that feed corn from South Dakota, for example, contained eleven times the selenium of a similar corn grown in Michigan.

Supplementation with 200 micrograms a day of selenium is considered safe and none of the patients in the cancer study showed any measurable signs of selenium toxicity. All, however, were from areas of the country where there are low levels of selenium in the soil.

Signs of selenium toxicity can begin to appear after a prolonged intake of 1,000-plus micrograms a day. The symptoms of selenium toxicity include a garlicky odor to the breath, sweat, and urine; a mottling of the teeth; loss of hair and nails; and skin lesions. To be prudent, it is always best to check with your physician.

The Carotenes: Carrot-Colored Compounds That Count

Studies looking for links between diet and disease consistently find that the incidence of killer diseases such as heart disease and certain cancers goes down as the consumption of vegetables (and fruits) increases. Over the years, scientists have been trying to learn what causes this "vegetable effect." Is it something in the vegetables themselves, or just the fact that the more vegetables you eat, the less room you might have for other, less healthy fare? The presence of a family of compounds called the carotenes is likely to be one of the answers.

One of the most common carotenes, beta-carotene, is related to vitamin A; in fact, it looks like two pieces of vitamin A stuck together. Whenever there's a need for vitamin A and beta-carotene is present, the body activates an enzyme that changes it into the active vitamin. But when a sufficient amount of vitamin A is present, beta-carotene and the other carotenes, are available to perform other functions, and this is where these compounds really begin to shine. Basically, when enough carotenes are present, they serve as antioxidants.

What does *antioxidant* mean? Obviously, we need oxygen to stay alive. But it turns out that oxygen, in the wrong place at the wrong time, can do serious damage to the body. The problem comes when the oxygen reacts with fats and forms "free radicals"—oxidized fats that damage cells and are believed to be involved in the development of heart disease, cancer, aging, and a host of other ailments.

Antioxidants present in the carotene family are able to stifle the production of compounds associated with an increased risk of disease.

How Much Is Enough?

Every day you should have no less than one serving of a food that's rich in carotenoids. You will find them in most dark green, yellow, and orange vegetables; particularly rich sources include yams, sweet potatoes, butternut squash, carrots, broccoli, kale, turnip greens, spinach, cabbage, mangoes, papaya, apricots, and cantaloupe.

Aiming for at least five servings of fruits and vegetables per day is the best way to ensure that your body is getting an ample amount of these important nutrients. (A typical serving is a medium piece of fruit, 1 cup of a leafy vegetable, 1/2 cup of fruit or cooked vegetables, 1/4 cup of dried fruit, or 6 ounces of a fruit or vegetable juice.)

I would stay away from foods made with *olestra*—especially if you have just eaten any carotene-containing foods. Research has shown that olestra has a distinct ability to grab on to carotenes and pull them out of the body before they can be absorbed.

The carotenes are essentially nontoxic. When you eat more than the body needs, the excess is removed naturally. Perhaps the most noticeable effect from a large intake is that you might actually begin to look like a carrot. The condition is most noticeable in fair-skinned people, and appears on the palms, the soles, and the center of the face. However, carotinemia, as it is called, is harmless, and the coloring will disappear when the intake of the carotenes is reduced. The coloring occurs because in addition to its nutritional qualities, carotenes are strong colorants. In fact, beta-carotene is used as a color additive in foods such as cheddar cheese, butter, and margarine—anywhere a natural orange color is desired.

Boning Up on Calcium

According to the most recent nutrition monitoring in the United States, most Americans do not get the calcium they need. When most of us think of the mineral calcium, we tend to think only of bones and teeth. There's logic to this, as 99 percent of the calcium in our body is in our bones and teeth. But aside from this well-known role, calcium also plays a key role in muscle contraction, blood coagulation, the immune system, blood pressure, and a blood-pressure-related complication of pregnancy called preeclampsia. A new wrinkle was added to calcium's résumé when a link was found between the taking of calcium supplements and a decreased risk of colon cancer.

The bones in our skeleton, despite their solid feel, are involved in a continuous process of mineral deposits and withdrawals. You could think of it just like a savings account. Childhood, adolescence, and early childhood—up to about age thirty—are the critical times to increase our calcium savings, as it is during these periods that the body has the greatest capacity to save dietary calcium. The amount of savings, however, depends entirely on the calcium in the diet, and the importance of this cannot be overemphasized.

Once we hit our thirties the body's automatic teller begins to shift gears. Our dietary deposits are no longer able to keep pace with the withdrawals, no matter how much calcium we eat. The third decade of life is the start of a slow but continuous erosion of the skeleton. From that point on, diet helps determine how fast this deterioration occurs.

The key weight-bearing bones in the body are the hip, upper thigh, and spine. If the mineral content of these bones dips too low, they lose their ability to support the body and can snap or begin to crumble without warning.

This condition is called osteoporosis (os-tee-oh pore-OH-sis). At present, osteoporosis is incurable. It's believed to account for well over a million broken bones every year and is indirectly involved in one in five deaths in people over seventy. It's estimated that one-third of the postmenopausal women in this country suffer from this disease.

Other factors besides a long-term low calcium intake that increase the risk of osteoporosis include being female, passing through menopause before age forty-five, a lack of weight-bearing physical activity, being underweight, being Caucasian, smoking, consuming excessive alcohol, and having a family history of the disease.

During pregnancy the demand for calcium increases dramatically. This makes sense as the mineral is needed not only for the mother's body, but to help construct the skeleton of the developing fetus.

Preeclampsia is a life-threatening condition during pregnancy that affects both mother and unborn child. It occurs in about 7 percent of pregnancies, usually during the second half of pregnancy, and is more common in first pregnancies, and in women under twenty-five or over thirty-five years of age. The symptoms of preeclampsia include headache, visual disturbances, nausea, vomiting, and abdominal pain. Having high blood pressure is a key risk factor for preeclampsia, as is having diabetes or any kidney disease.

A study in the *Journal of the American Medical Association* found that calcium supplements can lead to an important reduction in high blood pressure and life-threatening preeclampsia during pregnancy. The study relied on the taking of calcium supplements, but there is no reason to think it couldn't be done with food. This, in fact, might be preferable, as the body would then be getting a wider variety of the nutrients it needs. Whatever the method, though, greater attention to calcium is certainly needed.

Best Food Sources

Calcium can be found in many types of foods, but when dietary sources are discussed, milk and milk products tend to move center stage. Dairy products represent over 75 percent of the calcium in the American diet. One 8-ounce glass of skim milk contains about 302 milligrams of calcium; that's 25 percent of the RDA for a teenager or young adult. Milk products, however, are not the only source of calcium.

This is important to know because many people choose not to drink milk or can't tolerate dairy products because of either lactose intolerance or an allergy to milk. For lactose intolerance, there are remedies available. For a milk allergy, however, you will have to get calcium elsewhere. There are plenty of foods besides dairy that contain calcium. It is found in green leafy vegetables, small fish with edible bones, broccoli, dried fruits, legumes, and nuts. Other options include calcium-fortified foods, such as cereal or orange juice.

Calcium Sources

¹/₄ lb. sardines	433 mg
1 cup almonds	316 mg
1 cup arugula	302 mg
8 oz. calcium-fortified orange juice	302 mg
1 cup collard greens	304 mg
¹/₂ cup boiled amaranth	276 mg
1 cup cooked broccoli	180 mg
¹/₂ cup garbanzo beans	150 mg
¹/₄ pound tofu	150 mg
5 dried figs	144 mg
1 tbsp. blackstrap molasses	137 mg
¹/₂ cup cooked soybeans	102 mg
¹/₂ cup cooked navy beans	70 mg
¹/₂ cup dried apricots	67 mg

What About Calcium Supplements?

Another option is to take calcium in pill form. While this doesn't remedy a poor diet, it will provide the nutrients your body needs. Keep in mind that as with most minerals, calcium has to be in solution to be absorbed. Calcium carbonate, the most common and least expensive, is found in antacids such as Tums. This form, however, is the least soluble of the calcium salts. It requires an acid environment to dissolve and should be taken with meals or with a glass of orange or tomato juice.

Calcium citrate, calcium gluconate, and calcium lactate are more soluble, but they also cost considerably more. These compounds have less calcium per unit weight, so the pill size is larger than a comparable-strength calcium carbonate supplement.

One economical alternative is to purchase calcium carbonate powder by the pound (you may be able to get it through your local pharmacy or health food store). It is stable indefinitely at room temperature. Sprinkle about $1/8$ teaspoon of this white, tasteless powder on your food a few times a day; tomato-based sauces or other acid foods are ideal. Don't overdo it, though, or your food could taste gritty. One pound should last over a year.

> When considering calcium supplements, keep in mind that other nutrients, such as magnesium, vitamins A, B_6, and D, phosphorous, fluoride, and boron are needed for calcium absorption and healthy bones. Supplements should not be considered a remedy for a poor diet, but they can provide some of the nutrients your body needs.

6. Water:

The Forgotten Nutrient

For many it is the forgotten nutrient, but our bodies require more water than any other thing we ingest. We might survive for many weeks without food (if you call that living), but we would last only a few days without water. Despite this, perhaps because of its wide availability, water's importance as a nutrient is often overlooked.

Once inside our body, though, water intermingles with our vitamins, minerals, glucose, and amino acids to become the medium in which human life exists. All our chemical reactions take place in and around this vital fluid, and often water is an ingredient or product in these reactions.

A human embryo is approximately 97 percent water by weight. At birth the body is about 77 percent water, and by adulthood, it's down to around 60 percent. Water content varies according to gender and the respective amounts of bodily tissues. Muscle, for example, is about 75 percent water by weight, whereas adipose (fat) tissue is about 25 percent water. Even bones are more than 20 percent water by weight. This means that a muscular, heavy-boned individual tends to have a higher proportion of body water.

Water helps maintain the body's operating temperature. Those who live near a lake or ocean are familiar with the temperature-moderating effects that water can have on the environment. We also rely on this effect in our bodies. The water in our tissues helps to keep our body temperature relatively constant. This is important because essential organs, such as the brain, are sensitive to changes in temperature.

Aside from buffering the effects of climate, water also helps the body to release heat—that which is produced internally as a by-product of muscular work and biochemical activity. To make sure things don't get too hot, the body relies on evaporation, a process that uses up heat energy. The relief comes through exhaling water vapor through the lungs, or through the cooling effect of perspiration on the skin.

The articulating surfaces in our joints are "oiled" by water-based solutions. Our eyes are constantly bathed to keep the tissues moist and clean, and the digestive tract and lungs also experience the lubricating and cleansing effects of water.

Water is the transporter of supplies and by-products to and from various points in the body. Nutrients and other essentials are usually in water-soluble forms so that they can ride through the major fluid pathways to their various destinations. Water also dilutes toxins and waste materials, and helps usher them out of the body. Even those materials that don't dissolve in water, such as fats and cholesterol, have special water-based transport proteins (lipoproteins) that help shuttle them around the body.

The water in the body also functions as a shock absorber. A developing fetus is cushioned by the fluid environment of the uterus. The brain and spinal cord are also surrounded by water-based compartments that help shield these vital organs from concussion.

How Much Do We Need?

It's estimated that the body needs from 1 to 1.5 liters of water for every 1,000 Calories in our diet. This translates to a minimum of about eight 8-ounce glasses of water every day for the average person. Individuals who live in hot or dry climates are likely to need more, as are those who engage in physical exertion.

This water is essential because the wastes and toxins that accumulate as a natural course of metabolism can only be concentrated to a certain degree. Any excess salt we might have eaten has to be eliminated and the kidneys are only able to concentrate salt into water to a set degree. That's the reason why we can't survive on seawater—the concentration of salt is too high. The kidneys have to draw extra body water to purge the seawater's excess salt from our system.

Your daily fluid intake can come from drinking water or other beverages such as juice, milk, or soft drinks. Fruits and vegetables can also be counted, as they're about 80 percent water by weight. Don't count your intake of coffee, tea, or alcohol, though, as these have a diuretic (water-removing) effect that tends to cancel out their contribution.

How Safe Is Our Water?

In this country, access to fresh water is taken for granted. Now that we know more about the "why" and the "how much," we shouldn't ignore where our water is coming from. About 80 percent of the people in the United States rely on water from their municipal water supply; the remaining 20 percent use well water.

There are many factors that can affect the safety of your home water supply. If, for example, you live in an industrial area, there may be a risk of contaminants. If you live in an agricultural area, agricultural chemicals seeping into your ground water could be a problem. And even if the water coming into your house is pure, lead in your pipes or faucets could be releasing that dangerous heavy metal into the water you use.

Chlorine is another potential cause for concern. For more than seventy-five years, chlorine has been used to disinfect public water supplies. Chlorine is used in about 75 percent of the drinking water in this country. There's a possibility, however, that the chlorine itself may pose a health risk. Not only does chlorine kill the bacteria, it reacts with natural material and man-made pollutants to form compounds, such as chloroform, that are known carcinogens.

How can you determine whether there's a problem with your water? And if so, what do you need to do? You can start by requesting the annual report of water quality from the department that supplies the water to your house. The utility should be listed in your local Yellow Pages. If you decide to have your water tested, this is best done through an independent testing laboratory.

The Environmental Protection Agency (EPA) has a Safe Drinking Water hotline (1-800-426-4791) weekdays from 9 a.m. to 5:30 p.m. EST. The EPA will answer questions about the safety of the water supply, where to test water, and what to test for.

> There are plenty of home water-treatment devices on the market ranging in price from the tens to the thousands of dollars. But only after you learn more about the quality of your particular water supply can you decide if any purification is advised and, if so, which system would be best suited to your needs.

Specialty Water Glossary

Once you get past tap water, there's a sea of possibilities and prices.

Still Water

Mineral Water: Water that is drawn from an underground source that has at least 250 parts per million of dissolved mineral solids.

Artesian Water: Water that is drawn from a source that taps into a specific water-bearing rock formation in a confined area.

Spring Water: Water that naturally flows out of the ground. Spring water has no added minerals, nor can any minerals be taken away.

Natural Spring Water: Spring water collected without pumping or processing.

Hard Water: Water that contains higher levels of calcium and magnesium.

Soft Water: Water from which calcium and magnesium have been removed and replaced (usually) by sodium.

Drinking Water: Noncarbonated water with no guarantee that it comes from a particular source or has been given a special treatment.

Purified Water: Water from which minerals have been removed. (Also called demineralized, de-ionized, or distilled water.)

Distilled Water: The condensed steam of boiled water, a process that removes all minerals.

Deionized Water: Water from which minerals have been removed by a deionizer.

Water with Gas

Carbonated Water: Water to which carbon dioxide gas has been added under pressure.

Sparkling Water: The same as carbonated water.

Club Soda: Carbonated, filtered tap water with minerals added for taste. Can contain small amounts of caffeine or alcohol, so be sure to check the label.

Seltzer Water: Carbonated, filtered tap water that has no added minerals.

7. Understanding the Digestive System

The body likes things simple. Food, by contrast, is a complex combination of different types and sizes of nutrients and nonnutrient ingredients. In order for your body to absorb what foods contain, it first has to take them apart piece by piece. This assembly line, or should we say *dis*assembly line, is our digestive system.

The "workers" along your digestive tract are *enzymes*—chemicals with specific abilities to pull apart the proteins, carbohydrates, or fats in food. The digestive system is the epitome of specialization in that each of its enzymes can perform only one type of action on one type of nutrient. For example, one enzyme specializes in splitting big proteins into smaller pieces, but a different one is needed to complete the job. As a result, the normal digestive system requires over a dozen different enzymes to digest a typical meal. The beauty of the human digestive system is that it's specifically designed for a mixed diet. Different types of food are handled in specific areas. That's the reason we don't have to eat our foods one at a time.

Digestion, it turns out, starts even before we begin eating. When you're hungry, just thinking about food is enough to start the saliva running into your mouth, the fluids into your stomach, and to prime the muscles of the stomach for the meal about to head its way.

Saliva is mostly water, but it also contains enzymes that begin the work of breaking down carbohydrates. Giving each mouthful a good chew aids digestion because it mixes the food with saliva. This not only helps carbohydrate digestion, it makes the food easier to swallow through the esophagus and into the stomach.

Our muscular stomach churns the food into chyme, a liquid mass with a creamy consistency that then enters the small intestines. While in the stomach, food is exposed to strong digestive acids and enzymes. This causes the structure of food to crumble and prepares it for further digestion and absorption.

Carbohydrates tend to pass through the stomach quickest, followed by proteins and then fats, which take the longest to be released. The stomach protects itself from its own corrosive chemicals with a mucous layer that insulates it from the food being digested.

As the chyme departs the stomach, it is immediately doused with the body's own antacid solution. Your meal is now in the small intestines—a virtual enzyme factory where the main part of digestion and absorption takes place. Enzymes and other digestive aids produced in the liver, pancreas, and small intestines are unleashed upon the chyme in an orderly fashion. There are specific areas in the small intestines where different nutrients are absorbed. If all goes well, by the time your food reaches its respective absorptive surfaces, digestible carbohydrates have been broken down into simple sugars, proteins have been reduced to amino acids, and fats have been separated into individual fatty acids.

Vitamins and minerals don't require digestion, but to be absorbed by the body, they need to be separated from the food in which they came. Some vitamins and minerals are absorbed alone, but others have to be ushered in with a special carrier substance that's produced by the body and released into the digestive tract.

For example, the fat-soluble vitamins need to hook onto

a fatty acid to gain entrance. Vitamin B_{12} needs to link with a protein called "intrinsic factor," which is released by the stomach. And calcium and certain forms of iron have to find their respective "binding proteins" before they can be absorbed.

Fiber is unique in that the digestive system lacks the enzymes to break it down. As a result, the fiber in our food makes the complete trip from the mouth, through the stomach and small intestine, and into the large intestines. This undigested fiber adds to the bulk of the stool that is eventually eliminated from the body.

Once food enters the large intestine, which includes the colon and rectum, most digestion is over. The remaining task is to absorb water. This action prepares the undigested residue of the chyme for eventual elimination through the rectum.

The large intestine is not an empty tube, however; it is inhabited by a host of bacteria, called the intestinal flora, that live off the part of food our body does not absorb. Occasionally, food arriving in the large intestines includes carbohydrates that the body had trouble digesting. This might include some of the complex carbohydrates found in beans and other legumes, or the milk sugar (lactose) in those who have trouble digesting milk. When this happens, the intestinal flora devour these compounds and give off methane and other gases as a by-product. This can contribute to bloating and the production of gas, or flatus.

Flatulence Facts

Since foods affect people differently, any of a wide variety can appear on a particular person's "gas" list. Common culprits include dairy products, beans and other legumes, certain grains, cereals, vegetables, nuts, and seeds. Beans, lentils, and other legumes have a notorious reputation for gas because they contain a type of carbohydrate the body does not completely digest.

The gassy nature of foods, though, can even vary from meal to meal. For example, a large glass of skim milk or a bowl of beans on an empty stomach would probably produce more gas than the same serving eaten with a meal. This is explained by the slower rate at which a meal's combination of protein, fat, and carbohydrates travels through the digestive system. When it finally arrives at the large intestines, there's a mixture of materials to occupy the attention of the bacterial flora. On the other hand, when a single gassy food is eaten, the flora focus on the one, problem-causing material.

It's also known that some people tolerate large servings of foods that cause excessive gas in others. It's unclear how much of this is due to differences in digestive ability, how often we eat a particular food, or even such factors as whether we're relaxed or anxious, the speed at which we eat, or how completely we chew.

If you are constantly bothered by gas, start keeping a food diary. On the days your problem is most bothersome, make a note of the foods you have eaten, the meal conditions, and even your state of mind. Often a pattern emerges that can give you hints about ways to eat, methods of preparation, or more tolerable serving sizes. In addition, over-the-counter food supplements can help with a couple of the more troublesome carbohydrates. Lactase pills or drops supply the enzyme that digests the gas-causing lactose. Or you can simply drink lactose-reduced milk.

As with any physical complaint, discuss the situation with your health professional. Although food is usually the cause of flatulence, any digestive upset may be a reaction to medication or a sign of other problems that should be investigated more thoroughly.

Intestinal Flora:
The Benevolent Bugs Inside Us

Despite their reputation for causing infection and ill health, not all bacteria are problematic. In fact, there is a vast colony of "friendly" bacteria that live in the lower portion of the digestive system. These bacterial inhabitants are known as the intestinal flora, and they play an important role in our general health.

The lineup of potential benefits from healthy intestinal flora is nothing short of impressive. Research has associated these friendly bacteria with protection against colon cancer and other diseases in the intestines; protection against vaginal yeast infections; stimulation of the immune system; enhanced absorption of the protein, vitamins, and minerals in milk; and a reduction of the symptoms of lactose intolerance. In the large intestines, or colon, where the bacteria live, it's not all a one-sided affair. Alongside the friendly bacteria are other, not-so-friendly bugs seeking to gain the upper hand. Foods such as yogurt contain the types of benevolent bugs that can help strengthen the friendly flora and make it a stronger ally.

The use of yogurt and the history of bacteria in dairy products dates from the Bible. In those days, well before refrigeration, any attempt to store milk led to sour milk. At some point, it was discovered there were different types of sour milk and that only some made people ill.

With little understanding of how or why, people found that by taking a small amount from a "good" batch of sour milk and causing a similar souring in a new batch of fresh milk, they could store the milk for longer periods of time. In this way, the "culturing" of milk became an early form of food processing and preservation.

The notion that cultured dairy products might be healthful was popularized in 1906, when Elie Metchnikoff, a

Russian biologist working at the Pasteur Institute in Paris, proposed that health and longevity were linked to the type of bacteria living in the intestines. In his 1906 book, *The Prolongation of Life,* Metchnikoff attributed the health and long lives of Balkan tribes to the bacteria used to make the yogurt that was a staple of their diet.

The diet of the flora consists of the undigested/unabsorbed material in the foods we eat. Scientists have begun to study the factors that influence the bacteria in the intestinal flora. Researchers have discovered that although the flora is usually quite stable, it can be affected by what we eat and any medications we might take. Whenever there's a rapid change in the flora, there may be temporary discomforts such as cramps, diarrhea, bloating, or gas. The makeup of the flora will be affected by radical changes in our diet, such as the addition or removal of large amounts of fiber. Physical or emotional stress can also change the conditions of the lower intestines where the flora live. Some researchers speculate that the effect of stress on the intestinal flora might predispose the body to the diarrhea often experienced by travelers.

The key to any health benefits from intestinal flora is keeping the balance of power on the side of the benevolent bugs. This is not always an easy task, as there are thousands of strains of bacteria—both friendly and unfriendly—as well as several different yeast organisms.

Of all these factors, however, nothing affects the flora more than antibiotics. When taken to eliminate illness-causing bacteria, antibiotics destroy friend and foe alike, which permits yeast organisms normally kept in check by the friendly flora to grow in greater numbers. This is one reason why yeast infections often flare up during and after the taking of antibiotics.

One way to maintain a healthy flora is to keep sources of friendly bacteria, like yogurt or acidophilus milk, in your diet. Yogurt, although made from milk, is well tolerated by people with lactose intolerance—the reduced ability to digest the lactose in milk. This is because yogurt bacteria produce their own lactose-digesting enzyme.

To provide any of the additional health benefits, though, your source of friendly bacteria must contain a live, or active, culture. As the activity of friendly bacteria can decrease with age, it's best to eat yogurt that's as fresh as possible. In addition, some yogurt products are heat-treated, which kills off the bad as well as the good bacteria. (If a product is heat-treated, it has to say so on the label.)

The standard bacteria used to culture milk are *S. thermophilus* and *I. bulgaricus*. Some yogurt contains added *I. acidophilus* or *bifidus* bacteria. These types have special value because, unlike the standard yogurt bacteria, they are better equipped to establish themselves as long-term residents in the intestinal flora. Along the same line, milk drinkers should consider switching to low-fat milk with added *I. acidophilus*. For a few pennies more, you get all the potential benefits from this bacteria in every glass and there's no difference in taste.

Friendly Flora from Frozen Yogurt

Frozen yogurt is made from a specially formulated premix. Similar to cup yogurt, the premix is made from milk that has been cultured by a strain of friendly bacteria. Unlike yogurt in the cup, however, the culturing process is halted before the characteristic tartness can develop. The mix is then pasteurized—a step that kills potentially harmful bacteria along with the friendly bacteria used to culture the milk.

A number of manufacturers of frozen yogurt premix add a new batch of friendly bacteria after pasteurization. Because of this, their frozen yogurt can contribute to the health of intestinal flora. So if you're a frozen yogurt fan, it pays to find a brand that adds new culture after pasteurization. Ask at your frozen yogurt store, or read the label if you buy a packaged product.

Depending on the fat content of the yogurt, the premix will contain any of a variety of stabilizers, such as carrageen, guar gum, and carob bean gum. These are safe, naturally occurring substances that help reduce the formation of coarse ice crystals and, along with constant stirring by the yogurt dispensing machine, help maintain the dessert's characteristically smooth texture.

When compared with a flavored cup yogurt, most frozen yogurt contains comparable amounts of protein, carbohydrates, and calcium. Of course, this assumes that you don't pile on the sugary, high-fat crumbled candy bars, broken cookies, or sprinkles typically offered at the soft-serve yogurt counter.

Flora Supplements

Most natural and health food stores sell *I. acidophilus* and *bifidus* as a food supplement. These capsules, when taken as directed on a regular basis, can be an excellent nondairy source of the friendly flora. As with yogurt, though, freshness is important, so make sure you use it up before the expiration date.

Food Combining

The theory of food combining is based on the idea that the way foods are combined (or not combined) is the key to digestion and health. As this questionable theory goes, an easy-to-digest food, such as fruit, should never be eaten with proteins or fatty foods, which take longer to digest. To do so would delay the digestion of the fruit and allow the fruit sugar to ferment and putrefy. This, the theory concludes, would cause several health problems. Other forbidden combinations include starchy foods, such as bread or potatoes, together with protein foods, such as meat or fish.

There's no physical reason to believe the theory. The beauty of the human digestive system is that it's specifically designed for a mixed diet. The different types of foods in our diet each are handled in a specific region of the digestive system.

> Some people may find that certain foods or food combinations don't work for them. This is more a result of individuality than of a digestive defect of the human species. Barring your individual preferences, there is no physical necessity for refraining from including a variety of foods at every meal.

Do We Need Extra Enzymes from Food?

The line between science and sales promotion is often blurred, and the topic of enzymes is a good case in point. Enzymes are found throughout nature. They are needed to help break down foods for absorption and utilization. Seeds, for example, typically contain the makings of a new plant (germ) surrounded by a fat or carbohydrate energy source, be it fats or carbohydrate. When you water a seed, you trigger the seed's enzyme that breaks down the stored energy, allowing the plant to grow.

In our own bodies, enzymes help us make use of the energy in foods, but they're also needed to build complex substances and help transform one compound to another. A healthy body normally produces all the enzymes it needs. One defining characteristic of enzymes is that while they play a role in changing things around them, they, themselves, remain unchanged. The body produces its own assortment of digestive enzymes, and each one is specialized. The enzymes that digest starch, for example, cannot work on fat or protein.

There are a number of common situations in which extra enzymes might be used as a supplement. One example stems from the fact that a high proportion of adults no longer produces a sufficient amount of lactase, the enzyme that is needed to digest the carbohydrate lactose, found in milk. The symptoms of this "lactose intolerance" may include intestinal gas, cramping, and diarrhea. By taking lactase supplements along with a milk product, people can enjoy lactose-containing foods with any annoying side effects. Another popular enzyme supplement, called Beano, contains alpha-galactosidase, which is an enzyme that helps digest the carbohydrate found in beans and other vegetables.

Aside from these examples, there are also medical situations in which dietary enzymes might be prescribed. The pancreas produces the most of our digestive enzymes. If a medical problem develops that affects the pancreas's ability to either produce or deliver its enzymes to the digestive tract, the body will be unable to absorb a wide variety of essential nutrients. Individuals with such problems would need to take enzyme supplements, similar to the way that a diabetic needs to take insulin.

But what about those of us that don't have any specific enzyme-related malady? Could supplementary enzymes help us as well? This question shifts us away from established science to the gray area of unproven suppositions. There is a school of thought that holds that we derive special benefits from extra enzymes. The theory states that our life span is closely intertwined with our ability to produce enzymes. The idea is that we can only manufacture a fixed amount of enzymes, and as soon as we run out, the game, so to speak, is over.

Fresh fruits and vegetables, the theory continues, contain "live enzymes," which get deactivated by cooking. By eating a diet based around fresh, whole foods, or by taking enzyme supplements, we can effectively spare our body's enzymes and enable ourselves to live to a ripe old age.

There is little question that fresh, whole fruits and vegetables are among the most nutritious foods you can put in your body, but I have difficulty accepting this enzyme theory on face value—especially the part about the body having a fixed amount of enzymes. Fresh foods are healthful not because they contain enzymes, but because they are our richest source of nutrients. And then there's the fact that enzymes themselves are proteins. They will be inactivated in the acid environment of our stomach and then digested with all the other proteins we eat.

> We should eat and enjoy fresh, whole foods, but we should not cherish them for any special enzyme powers. Think of them as being the nutrient-rich foods that they are. Unless you have a specific digestive problem, the taking of supplementary enzymes is a questionable proposition.

PART II

From Nutrition Theory to the Real World

8. Using Food to Fight Heart Disease

The war against heart disease is not going well. There has been some progress, in that fewer people are dying, but the prevalence of the nation's number-one killer disease remains virtually unchanged. Optimistic statistics may be nothing more than a reflection of improved methods of diagnosis and medical treatment.

The reason for the lack of progress is as simple as it is profound: *We are not focused on the real problem.* The American public has been persuaded to wear blinders that only let them see the fat and cholesterol in their diet, and the cholesterol level in their blood, as the key factors causing heart disease. Following this line of thought, it then follows that all one has to do is to reduce the fat and cholesterol in their diet, and like magic, the risk of heart disease will dance out of their life. Well folks, it isn't that simple. There's little question that fat and cholesterol play a role in heart disease, but they are not the unqualified culprits we've been led to believe.

Heart disease results when there's a blockage preventing blood flow through the arteries. If these vessels service the heart muscle, it can lead to a heart attack, and if a blockage from any artery gets loose and travels to the brain, it can lead to a stroke. Such blockages often begin as a kind of scratch, or lesion, on the inner lining of the artery. Because the failure of a blood vessel can be life-threatening, after such an injury is detected, the body immediately takes steps to repair the damage and wall off the affected area. Cholesterol is one of the key ingredients in this repair process.

You can think of cholesterol as being part of the "plaster" that the body uses to repair the injuries to its blood vessels. The amount of cholesterol "blockage" in our blood vessels depends, in part, upon the level of injury to the tissues. And as damage to blood vessels increases, so too does the level of cholesterol in our blood. Most of the cholesterol in the body is manufactured in the liver. When cholesterol is present in the foods we eat, the liver is programmed to make less.

Cholesterol has many important functions in the body. It's a waxy substance that does not dissolve in our water-based blood. As such, it has to be shuttled around the blood inside fat-carrying proteins called lipoproteins. There are four basic types of lipoproteins, but two appear to play important roles in heart disease. The first, called low-density lipoproteins (LDL), can be thought of as the carrier of cholesterol into general circulation. The second, called high-density lipoprotein (HDL), shuttles cholesterol on its way out of the body. As the proportion of blood cholesterol traveling in the LDLs goes up, so does your risk of heart disease. By contrast, as the cholesterol in the HDLs goes up, your risk decreases. Because of this, it's convenient to think of LDLs as the "least desirable" and HDLs as the "highly desirable" forms of cholesterol.

The level of LDLs tends to be high in developing heart disease, because LDL is the carrier for cholesterol when it's on its repair missions.

As you can tell from this scenario, cholesterol is not the responsible party; it's only present as a symptom of the problem. Thus, our continued focus on cutting cholesterol out of the diet and lowering blood cholesterol as ends in themselves may help explain why our efforts against heart disease are going so poorly.

Oxidized Fats: The True Culprits

The real villains in heart disease are those agents responsible for blood-vessel damage in the first place. It now looks as though the main source of this damage has to do with oxygen and its tendency to react (oxidize) with fatty substances such as fats and cholesterol. These "oxidized fats" tend to combine with whatever is nearby and can damage the lining of the blood vessels—the first step down the road to heart disease. Scientists have discovered that oxidized fats are directly responsible for the lesions that initiate the artery-clogging buildups.

Diet for a Healthy Heart

Once you accept the fact that fats are vulnerable to oxidation, it becomes clear why cutting back on dietary fat has some merit. It can decrease the amount of fats circulating in your bloodstream that might be susceptible to oxidation. But while low fat is an answer, it's not the only answer. The body has a two-pronged defense system to protecting itself from oxidation-related damages. The first helps prevent fats from being oxidized, and the second neutralizes those fats that have already had their deleterious dose of oxygen. These defenses, however, depend on a daily supply of nutrient-rich foods. The key is a diet that focuses on fruits, vegetables, legumes, and whole grains. The bottom line is that diets high in these nutrient-rich foods don't have to be overly restrictive in total fat so long as there aren't too many calories.

Heart-healthy diets should focus on monounsaturated oils, such as olive oil and be low in saturated and partially hydrogenated fats, as these have been shown to unnaturally increase the number of cholesterol-carrying LDLs in the bloodstream—a step that can stimulate the development of cholesterol blockages.

Finally, it is important to avoid eating fats that have

already been oxidized. Dietary sources of oxidized fats include those foods containing rancid fats, ones fried in overused unsaturated oils, and cholesterol-containing dried-food products, such as powdered eggs.

> Keep in mind that the fatty buildups that lead to heart disease can take decades to develop. When you cut back on dietary fat and cholesterol you only do a small part of the job. Of primary importance is the need to give your body the nutrients it needs to protect itself. This is just as—if not more—essential. This approach can make the difference between a continued stalemate and a forward offensive in the war against heart disease.

Don't Forget Fiber and Physical Activity

A considerable body of research evidence has accumulated that links an increased fiber intake (25 to 30 grams a day) with reduction in the risk of heart disease. And finally, a program of regular physical activity will also help out. (If you have been inactive, you should check with your physician before starting on any exercise program.)

Vitamin E and Heart Disease

One of the greatest dilemmas in the fields of health and nutrition is the uneasy balance between a scientist's need to establish safety and reliability, and people who want their "cures" now. Case in point: vitamin E.

Research published in the *New England Journal of Medicine* (NEJM) fueled an ongoing debate over whether a balanced diet can supply all one needs for optimal health. These particular results came from separate ongoing studies with 87,245 female nurses and 39,910 male health professionals. In both, the participants filled out questionnaires about their dietary habits and the supplements they took. At the onset of the studies, the women, aged thirty-four to sixty-nine, and men, aged forty to seventy-five, were free of any diagnosed heart disease.

The health statistics collected over the years revealed a significant relationship between the use of vitamin E supplements and a reduced risk of heart disease. In both studies, those with an intake of at least 100 International Units (IU) a day had a 40 percent lower risk of developing heart disease. The recommended daily allowance (RDA) for vitamin E is 15 IU for adult men and 12 IU for adult women.

These studies are only a small sample of the research evidence attesting to vitamin E's beneficial effect on the risk of heart disease. But the fact that such strong results came from a large group of people followed over many years is indeed impressive.

How Does Vitamin E Do It?

Vitamin E's main role is that of an antioxidant, and as such it helps to prevent free radicals from harming the tissues of your body. Free radicals are believed to be involved in the aging process and in the development of a host of ailments including heart disease and cancer. But the free radicals can be stopped in their tracks by an antioxidant such as vitamin E, which acts like a scavenger, attracting and reacting with wayward free radicals before they can cause any damage.

It turns out that one is hard pressed to design a diet high enough in vitamin E by relying only on food. Vitamin E is used in nature to protect plant seed oils, the energy source used by the developing seed to sprout, send down its roots, and grow to the point that it can begin producing energy on its own. That's why we find the highest concentrations of vitamin E in foods like seeds, nuts, and wheat germ.

Among vegetables, kale and sweet potatoes are the best sources. Aside from these natural food sources, you can always get your Recommended Daily Allowance (RDA) through a vitamin-fortified cereal.

The fact that vitamin E is most plentiful in fats can make it difficult for those on a low-fat diet. To get up to the 100 IUs—considered the minimum risk-reducing amount in the studies—one would have to pay an inordinate amount of attention to this nutrient.

Should You Take a Supplement?

To supplement or not to supplement is a difficult question to answer as vitamin E is not the end-all of a healthy diet. In an editorial accompanying the NEJM reports, caution was urged. It was pointed out that studies on the possible long-term side effects from vitamin E supplementation have not yet been conducted. This being said, however, doses up to 1,000 IU are generally considered safe for most people.

The scientific community is somewhat divided on the topic of vitamin E supplements, with respected researchers on both sides of the line. In my opinion the case in favor of vitamin E supplements is overwhelming. I've been taking about 400 IU a day for over twenty years, ever since I first began reading about vitamin E. Regardless of your decision, however, a healthy diet must remain your primary focus.

Adult Weight and Heart Disease

The tendency to carry extra weight is an unwelcome, yet all-too-common phenomenon of getting older—it's even OK'd by Uncle Sam. The 1990 height–weight tables put out by the U.S. Department of Agriculture and the U.S. Department of Health and Human Services feature a significant jump in the range of acceptable weights for adults when they enter the "over thirty-five years of age" category. That jump, however, may come with a stiff tariff in the form of an increased risk of heart disease.

A 1995 study in the *Journal of the American Medical Association* (JAMA) revealed that we should be paying more attention to how much weight we gain. It was discovered that even a moderate weight gain will significantly increase the risk of heart disease in middle-aged women despite the fact that their weight remains within established guidelines. The weight ranges of the "over thirty-five" category may be providing a false sense of security to those who have gained.

The JAMA study, performed at the Harvard School of Public Health, set out to assess the validity of the 1990 suggested weight guidelines. These guidelines express normal adult weights according to two age groups: nineteen to thirty-four, and thirty-five and older, and they appear to condone a significant weight gain as one reaches thirty-five years of age.

To test the guidelines, the scientists designed a "prospective cohort study," in which a specific group, or cohort, was selected and then followed for a number of years. The group, in this case, was 115,818 female registered nurses living in the United States, aged thirty to fifty-five in 1976, when the study began.

The JAMA study noted the volunteers' recall of what they weighed at eighteen years of age. For the fourteen-year study period, the scientists recorded the volunteers' changing weight patterns in tandem with the incidence of coronary heart disease, which was defined as either fatal or nonfatal heart attacks.

Studies such as these cannot predict with certainty, but they are good at summarizing the odds, referred to as the "relative risk," that an event—in this case, heart disease—will occur. In interpreting these results, keep in mind that a 100 percent relative risk is the same as "even odds," which is the same as saying no effect.

Height–Weight Tables

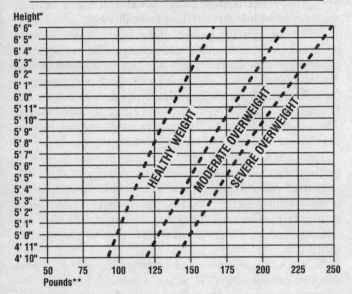

*Without shoes.

**Without clothes. The higher weights apply to people with more muscle and bone, such as many men. Source: USDA Report of the Dietary Guidelines Advisory Committee on the Dietary Guidelines for Americans, 1995, pages 23–24.

Taking the weight at eighteen years of age as the baseline, the study found that a gain of eleven to seventeen pounds carried with it a relative risk of 125 percent; a gain of eighteen to twenty-four pounds had a 164 percent relative risk; a gain of twenty-four to forty-three pounds had a relative risk of 192 percent (*note:* almost two to one odds of getting heart disease!); and an increase over forty-three pounds had a relative risk of 265 percent.

As you can see, weight gain is the key. It's unclear

Suggested Weight for Adults
(1990 U.S. Dept. of Agriculture and U.S. Dept. of Health and Human Services)

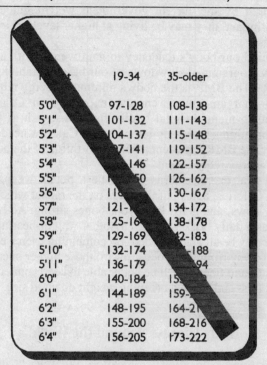

Height	19-34	35-older
5'0"	97-128	108-138
5'1"	101-132	111-143
5'2"	104-137	115-148
5'3"	97-141	119-152
5'4"	146	122-157
5'5"	50	126-162
5'6"	118	130-167
5'7"	121-	134-172
5'8"	125-16	138-178
5'9"	129-169	42-183
5'10"	132-174	-188
5'11"	136-179	94
6'0"	140-184	15
6'1"	144-189	159-
6'2"	148-195	164-21
6'3"	155-200	168-216
6'4"	156-205	173-222

Don't rely on tables that show suggested weights by age

whether it's the weight itself that poses the risk, or if it's the poor eating habits or decreased physical activity that often precedes and accompanies the weight gain. These factors were not considered.

It's also important to remember that this study only considers heart disease. There's a good rationale for this, though, because every year, almost twice as many women die from heart disease and stroke as from all forms of cancer combined.

The bottom line is that many women are being falsely reassured by the current government weight guidelines when, in fact, they may be living at higher levels of avoidable risk.

Behind our body's tendency to gain weight with age is the preprogrammed slowdown of our basal metabolic rate (BMR). The BMR is the body's minimum energy requirement—that amount of energy (expressed in Calories) needed to maintain vital bodily functions such as heart rate, breathing, and body temperature. Calories needed to satisfy the BMR represent a hefty two-thirds of the body's daily energy requirement.

Physical exercise turns out to be a potent weapon; it burns Calories, helps put the skids on the rate at which the BMR slows, and helps keep your bones strong. Activities such as a daily brisk walk or any other weight-bearing exercise may be all that's needed. By combining exercise with a shift away from fatty foods toward those higher in carbohydrates and fiber, you'll be better able to keep your energy needs high and cut that creeping weight down to size.

Heart Disease Around the World

Location . . . location . . . location. What works in real estate also rings true for one's blood cholesterol level and risk of heart disease.

A 1995 study in the *Journal of the American Medical Association* (JAMA) contained a follow-up to a landmark study referred to as the Seven Countries Study. The initial research provided extensive evidence about the international relationship between fat intake, blood cholesterol, and coronary heart disease (CHD). A key finding from that study was how Mediterranean countries consumed higher levels of dietary fat but did not experience the same risk of CHD as in the U.S. and Northern Europe. Now, in this follow-up study, scientists have attempted to explain this disparity. The findings have particular importance to us in America as our dietary miscues help make CHD the nation's number-one killer disease.

The original study looked at 12,773 men, forty to fifty-nine years of age, in the United States, Northern Europe (Finland), the Netherlands, Italy, Greece, Yugoslavia (now Serbia and Croatia), and Japan. Information about risk factors, such as smoking, diet, and high blood pressure, and a baseline blood cholesterol level was taken between 1958 and 1964 and at five- and ten-year intervals thereafter. Mortality statistics were then collected on the population for twenty-five years.

The data revealed cholesterol levels ranging from 160 to 170 mg/dL in the Japanese, up to 240 to 260 mg/dL in the U.S. and Northern Europe groups. Mortality from CHD ranged from 3 percent in the Japanese up to 20 percent in the Northern Europe group.

As an indication of the importance of location, the same cholesterol level represented a different CHD risk according to where you live. With a cholesterol level of 210 mg/dL, for example, mortality varied from 4 to 5 percent in Japan and the Southern Mediterranean, up to 12 percent in the United States, and 15 percent in Northern Europe.

Even a "safe" cholesterol level, such as 190 mg/dL, carried with it twice the risk of CHD mortality in Northern Europe as did the same level in the Mediterranean.

The explanation for this disparity involves the foods we eat and how they help determine whether our body can handle its dietary fat in a way that doesn't contribute to disease.

We have learned how fats have an ability to turn into free radicals when they combine with oxygen in the wrong place at the wrong time. We have also learned how these compounds are thought to trigger a chain reaction that sends us down the road to heart disease, cancer, certain forms of arthritis, aging, and a host of other ailments. It's a serious problem and one that's at the core of America's misguided way of eating. How, then, do we explain cultural eating patterns that have succeeded in marrying high-fat cuisine with a better state of health?

In recent decades we have discovered how the body is not without its defenses. There are antioxidant compounds in fresh fruits, vegetables, and grains that can stifle fat's destructive breakdown before serious damage can occur. Data from the Seven Countries Study and the follow-up reported in JAMA show that those living in Mediterranean Southern Europe have significantly higher intakes of fruit and vegetable antioxidants, such as beta-carotene, vitamin E, and the flavonoids.

In addition, the main food fat in the Mediterranean is olive oil, which is monounsaturated, whereas in the U.S. we consume more saturated and partially hydrogenated fat, and polyunsaturated oil, a combination that tends to be much more susceptible to disease-promoting oxidation.

The JAMA article points out that bringing down one's elevated blood cholesterol, as an end in itself, is not the optimum way to bring about significant reductions in the risk of CHD mortality. At present, it's not uncommon for persons with an elevated cholesterol value to be placed on cholesterol-lowering medications as their sole medical intervention. They may think they've found the answer to their problem if the drugs manage to bring down their cholesterol level, but what we're learning is that this approach does not get to the "heart" of the problem.

The study findings also have implications for today's growing variety of fat-free processed foods. An all-too-common remedy to an unbalanced, high-fat diet is to feast on a box of fat-free snack food. While this may cut your fat intake, it does little to help reduce your risk of heart disease.

Overall, a good, balanced diet, with its daily dose of

health-promoting nutrients, is one of the most effective antidisease strategies you could find.

Healthful Diets Around the World

• Low-fat cuisines, such as that of Japan, tend to have the best health statistics because in addition to low levels of fat, they include high amounts of vegetables, fruits, and high-fiber grains.

• *Healthful* higher-fat cuisines, such as those found in the Mediterranean, manage to strike a balance between rich foods and a daily intake of nutrient-rich, fresh vegetables, fruits, and high-fiber grains.

• *Contrast this with our society where we eat high fat AND fail to include those foods our body needs to maintain its health.*

---

9. The Menu for Long Life

Does good nutrition wield special powers to combat the aging process? Aging doesn't happen suddenly, in that you're young one day and old the next. Rather, it is a cumulative process that proceeds at different rates in different people. But diet and other lifestyle factors *can* play a central role in defining how that process will be expressed in your life.

This is a timely topic, considering that the baby-boom generation is now entering its fifth decade, and by the year 2020, over half the people in the United States will have joined the over-fifty crowd. The definition of what it means to be older, however, continues to undergo radical changes. Larger segments of the population are living longer, doing more, and enjoying better health than ever before.

Besides the obvious visible signs, the body's metabolism goes through radical change as it gets older. Research has shown that seniors may not be that efficient at regulating their food intake. One study, published in the *Journal of the American Medical Association,* took place at the USDA Nutrition Research Center on Aging at Tufts University. It looked at thirty-five men of normal weight; approximately half were young adults in their twenties and others were seniors between sixty-two and eighty years of age. For three weeks all the volunteers were fed a balanced diet, except that half the men in each group were underfed by 800 Calories a day and the other half were overfed by 1,000 Calories a day. After this period the men were allowed to eat whatever they wanted. The young adults adjusted their intakes, those who had been underfed ate more, and those who had been overfed ate less. The senior men, however, continued to eat in the same way.

Generally, an older body requires fewer Calories because it needs less dietary energy. In addition, the body may digest and absorb needed nutrients less efficiently. The ability to feel thirst may also diminish, resulting in an inadequate water intake. It's also common for older people to experience such diet-related problems as difficulty in chewing and a decreased sense of smell and taste.

Other problems, such as reduced vision, loss of mobility, loneliness, depression, and income limitations, may affect an individual's ability to partake of and enjoy the eating experience. Often, despondency over the loss of a partner affects the very desire to have a meal. All of these can lead to dramatic changes in what, how, and when people eat. The end result can be a diet that is lacking in key nutrients. Two examples are protein and vitamin D.

Protein in the Elderly

Surveys have shown that a large proportion of the elderly eat below the adult recommended dietary allowance (RDA) for protein, with the lowest amount being consumed by the homebound elderly. Such surveys went almost unnoticed because the levels involved weren't very far below the RDA.

One study took place at the metabolic ward of the U.S. Department of Agriculture's Human Nutrition Research Center on Aging at Tufts University in Boston. The study, published in the *American Journal of Clinical Nutrition,* involved twelve men and women fifty-six to eighty years of age. The volunteers lived at the facility twenty-four hours a day during the study. Although twelve volunteers are a small number for a study, "metabolic ward" research is very powerful because the scientists are able to control key factors, such as physical activity and adherence to the experimental diet, that otherwise might influence a study's results. The volunteers received two separate diets, one with protein at the RDA level, the other with protein at twice the RDA.

The data showed that the elderly volunteers weren't getting enough protein when fed at the current adult RDA level. This wasn't the case when they received twice the RDA amount.

Depending on the length and degree, there is a range of symptoms associated with an ongoing protein deficiency. (If the deficiency is severe enough, it can lead eventually to death.)

The dilemma is that these symptoms, which include increased susceptibility to disease, poor wound healing, fatigue, anemia, hair and skin problems, mental confusion, pallor, digestive disturbances, muscle wasting, and weight loss, are the very symptoms typically associated with aging. New information raises serious questions as to whether a chronic protein deficiency may be contributing to the decline of the elderly more than was previously thought.

The key with protein, however, is to have enough but not too much. Going overboard is not the answer. The typical high-protein American diet may be contributing to high incidence of osteoporosis in our society, because chronic protein excess can prevent dietary calcium from being absorbed. Have enough, but not too much. The adult protein requirement is about 11 grams of protein for every 30 pounds of ideal body weight (see chapter 1). Those over sixty years of age should count about 15 grams of protein per 30 pounds of body weight.

Vitamin D

Vitamin D is different from other essential nutrients in that, aside from being able to absorb it from food, our body is able to make this vitamin its own. Essential to the formula, however, are the ultraviolet rays of the sun.

A study in the *Journal of the American Medical Association* revealed how a lack of sunlight combines with poor nutrition and age-related changes in skin and kidney function to leave the homebound elderly at significant risk for a vitamin D deficiency.

The JAMA study looked at 244 volunteers; 116 had been confined indoors for at least six months, and the remaining 128 controls lived in a nursing home but were able to go out (free-living). All volunteers lived in Baltimore and were sixty-five to ninety-four years of age. Food intake was recorded and vitamin D levels were measured in the blood. The study did not include any volunteers on a medication or with a condition that might interfere with the level of vitamin D in the body.

When the data were examined it was found that the blood levels of vitamin D in the homebound were significantly lower than those who were free-living. More than half the sunlight-deprived elderly had blood levels indicating a vitamin D deficiency. Part of the difference could be explained by the fact that 83 percent of the homebound, as opposed to 36 percent of the free-living elderly, had vitamin D intakes below recommended levels.

One of vitamin D's main functions is to help the body absorb dietary calcium and phosphorous. Both of these minerals are needed to help make strong bones. Symptoms of a vitamin D deficiency are similar to those of a calcium deficiency—namely, an improper bone formation and increased rate of bone loss.

A lack of vitamin D will eventually give rise to "rickets,"

a deficiency disease that was prevalent in the 1600s during the industrial revolution in England. People had migrated from farms to the cities and while few were homebound, the smoke-filled air and high-rise apartments effectively blocked exposure to the sun.

In the early 1800s, cod-liver oil gained fame as an effective folk remedy against rickets, but it wasn't until 1922 that scientists at Johns Hopkins identified the compound responsible. First called the "calcium-depositing vitamin," it eventually became known as vitamin D. The recognition of the essential role of vitamin D in the absorption of calcium led to the recommendation that babies be given some source of the vitamin, such as cod-liver oil. In the 1930's the government began a fortification program that added vitamin D to milk, effectively eliminating the incidence of childhood rickets in this country.

The problems associated with a vitamin D deficiency, however, are now visiting our elderly. A vitamin D deficiency represents a special hazard for seniors struggling to stave off osteoporosis, the weak-bone disease that plagues those in their later years. A long-term deficiency of vitamin D can lead to osteomalacia, or "adult rickets," a condition that has many of the same symptoms as osteoporosis. A vitamin D deficiency can also contribute to general weakness and a rheumatoid-like pain in the lower extremities.

Although the body can make its own vitamin D upon exposure to sunlight (or a sunlamp), the process can be blocked by anything that blocks the sun. This applies to physical barriers such as a tree, a building, or a wide-brimmed hat, as well as ones less obvious such as a pane of glass, smoke, smog, or slathering on a high-powered sunscreen. Today's increased prevalence of skin cancer has led many to avoid exposure to the sun. This being the case, the elderly have to pay special attention to getting vitamin D from their diet.

Aside from its presence in supplements, good food

sources for vitamin D include fatty fish, such as salmon and tuna, egg yolk, liver, dairy products, and vitamin D-fortified foods, such as cereals, breads, and certain beverages.

One final word of caution: As with protein, it is important to not overdo it. Vitamin D can be toxic when taken to excess. The recommended intake for vitamin D is 400 International Units per day and toxicity symptoms have been reported with levels as low as four times this amount.

Practical Strategies

Studies have documented the importance of staying well-nourished as you age. One study, for example, showed that even among older people in good health, those whose diets contained more of the essential nutrients performed better on memory and learning tests. Good long-term eating habits also help out when you're ill. The payoff includes faster wound healing, fewer surgical complications, and shorter hospital stays.

One widely held theory of aging explains how the compounds called free radicals cause damage to the cells of the body. Free-radical damage has been associated with heart disease, cataracts, and certain types of cancer as well as other diseases of old age. Research has shown that a few nutrients, including vitamin E, vitamin C, beta-carotene, selenium, and zinc, have the ability to combat free-radical damage.

The best basic dietary advice remains to eat as wide a variety of healthy foods as possible. Eating the same foods day after day is unwise because it limits exposure to the different nutrients. Here are some other nutritional guidelines:

- Focus on fresh vegetables and fruits, low-fat dairy products, lean meats, nuts and seeds, legumes, and whole grains.
- When cooking, keep nonfat dry milk powder nearby

and sprinkle it in your food; it's a great source of protein, calcium, and vitamin D.

- Take advantage of the salad bars at supermarkets and restaurants; it's a great way to put together a nutritious meal without waste.

- Make a point to drink at least six to eight glasses of water or water-based beverages daily.

- If, for any reason, you cannot or will not eat a healthy diet, consider taking a vitamin/mineral supplement. While it's always preferable to get these nutrients from food, this may not be possible. The bottom line: It's better to get the nutrients from a supplement than not at all.

- If you decide you need a supplement, check with your physician beforehand about the effects it might have on any existing health conditions or prescription medications. Ask if you might benefit from additional amounts of certain vitamins or minerals. When shopping for a supplement, look for an inexpensive one-a-day type that contains minerals as well as vitamins. Take it with a meal to ensure better absorption.

Stay away from anti-aging gurus who promise longevity through their products and services—usually at a hefty price. Health fraud is big business, and older Americans make up about 40 percent of all victims. Don't become a statistic by joining this group, which wastes approximately $2 billion every year on fake anti-aging remedies.

Age-Related Weight Gain

The body's tendency to gain weight with age stems from a preprogrammed slowdown in its basal metabolic rate (BMR).

The BMR is the body's minimum energy requirement—that amount of energy (expressed in Calories) needed to maintain vital bodily functions, such as heart rate, breathing, and body temperature. Calories needed to satisfy the BMR represent a hefty two-thirds of the body's daily energy requirement.

The BMR begins to rise at birth and reaches its peak during childhood. After that, it decreases at a rate of about 2 to 4 percent per decade. The rate of decrease is affected by changes in the amount of muscle in the body. This is because muscle is an "active" energy-burning tissue, whereas body fat is an "inactive" energy-storage depot. Therefore, as activity decreases with age (a typical pattern), the decline of the BMR accelerates.

Repeated dieting can also decrease the BMR. Because a small amount of muscle tissue is lost during rapid weight loss, each episode of weight loss and regain leaves the body with a higher percentage of fat tissue. Cutting back on food is not the best, and certainly not the only, way to slow age-related weight gain. If not done with care, continual cutbacks could leave your diet lacking the full complement of essential nutrients.

Physical exercise turns out to be a more potent weapon; not only does the activity burn Calories, but it helps put the skids on the rate at which the BMR slows down and helps keep your bones strong. Activities such as a daily brisk walk or any other weight-bearing exercise may be all that's needed. By combining exercise with a shift away from fatty foods toward those higher in carbohydrates and fiber, you'll be better able to keep your energy needs high and cut that creeping weight down to size.

10. The Food–Mood Connection

The nutrients in our diet can influence whether we are alert, depressed, or ready to doze. Although the connections between what we eat and our levels of alertness aren't fully understood, it's fascinating to think that diet might help or hinder the way the brain works.

The idea of a link between diet and behavior came from studies on nutritional deficiencies. One of the first connections had to do with niacin, a water-soluble vitamin. In the early 1900s, as many as half the patients in hospitals for the insane in the southern United States were victims of a disease called pellagra (pe-LAY-gruh). Symptoms included skin rash, intestinal problems, and mental confusion that eventually led to insanity. At the time, diets among the poor living in the Southeast consisted primarily of cornmeal, salt pork, and molasses. This diet was deficient in protein and niacin as well as many other vitamins. In 1937, scientists discovered that pellagra was caused by a niacin deficiency. When a large dose of niacin was given to the pellagra victims, their insanity, as well as their other symptoms, disappeared like magic.

We now have a better understanding of the major deficiency diseases and their effect on behavior. Today, interest in this area has shifted toward looking at ways our diet might affect the way healthy individuals feel and perform.

It's been reported that skipping meals, especially breakfast, can have a negative effect on the way students perform in the classroom and on tests. Having too much to eat can also decrease alertness. One Scottish study showed that a large meal, such as the size often eaten during Thanksgiving, decreased performance on a complex task to about the same degree as going without sleep for a night. Additionally, although simple sugars are sources of quick energy, studies of adults show that high-carbohydrate meals often lead to sleepiness, decreased attention span, and impaired concentration.

Although no diet can counteract the tedium of repetitive tasks, what you eat can help determine whether you're awake on the job or ready to fall asleep. We know, for example, that large meals and those high in sugar or fat encourage drowsiness.

The tired feeling comes on in three stages. First, as you're eating, the pattern of blood flow begins to shift away from the muscles and toward the digestive tract in preparation to receive the nutrients from the food. Next, as sugar from the meal enters the bloodstream, insulin is released by the pancreas. These events favor the production of one of our brain's homemade tranquilizers, and we find ourselves gently persuaded to sit back and relax.

One reason behind this is that the body is unable to do a good job on digestion and on muscular work at the same time. The warning to not engage in vigorous swimming soon after a meal is based on this principle. But while such involuntary relaxation might be welcomed after a long day of work, it can be a real nuisance at ten a.m. or two p.m. Often, however, we encourage this by what we eat.

The day begins with a coffee-and-pastry breakfast. The caffeine plus the rapidly absorbed sugar provides an immediate energy surge. But as insulin is released, energy dwindles into the doldrums, and in a couple of hours you're ready to lay your head down on the desk. Then, low and behold, it's time for a coffee break; time for the snack machine and another jolt of java and it's up again for the next ride on the energy roller coaster.

If this cycle sounds too familiar, shift to smaller meals of complex carbohydrates and protein. For breakfast this could be a whole-grain, unsweetened cereal with low-fat or skim milk. If a sweetener is needed, opt for fruit over table sugar. Fructose, the carbohydrate found in most fruits, is not absorbed as quickly as sucrose and it doesn't have the same insulin-stimulating effect. By this same logic, fruits and raw vegetables, such as apples, oranges, and carrots, make excellent selections for the coffee break. Small, protein-based meals may actually encourage alertness and better performance. Certain amino acids in a protein meal encourage the brain to produce its own form of chemical stimulant.

Food's Effect on the Brain

The brain makes use of chemical substances named *neurotransmitters* that influence our level of alertness or relaxation. Two alertness neurotransmitters are dopamine and norepinephrine. When we eat protein, the food gets broken apart into its individual amino acids during digestion. One of these amino acids, tyrosine, can go into the brain and be used to help manufacture dopamine and norepinephrine.

Serotonin is one of the relaxation neurotransmitters. When carbohydrates are consumed, our blood sugar level tends to rise, which then causes the hormone insulin to be released by the pancreas. When this occurs, it encourages another amino acid, named tryptophan, to enter the brain. Tryptophan is used by the brain to form serotonin. This helps explain why some individuals feel lethargic after having a sugary snack on an empty stomach.

Although everybody may not react the same way, this simple model helps to explain why a meal based primarily on carbohydrates is likely to make us feel relaxed, while one that is based on protein—with or without some carbohydrate—can encourage alertness.

Sugar and Hyperactivity in Children

Many parents believe that sugar leads to hyperactive behavior in their children. To date, however, scientists have been unable to affirm any connection between sugar intake and hyperactivity.

In typical studies, children classified as "sugar responders" received either a sugared or an artificially sweetened beverage. Their behavior then was rated by their parents or scientists who were unaware of which treatment was being administered. Most studies have been unable to find an effect. In 1987, the Sugar Task Force of the U.S. Food and Drug Administration concluded that sugar was not linked to behavioral changes in children. This being said, however, it is reasonable to expect some children will be "recharged" after eating a sugary snack—particularly if they have been active and without food for a period of time. The simple sugars found in snack foods include glucose, corn syrup, honey, and table sugar. These carbohydrates are rapidly absorbed and cause the blood-sugar level to rise—key elements in the ability to affect behavior.

Nutrition for a Stressful Lifestyle

Whether it comes from the demands of family, a troubled relationship, a high-pressure job, or no job at all, stress is an all-too-common fact of life. And although good nutrition can help the body withstand day-to-day pressures, food and stress, it turns out, make a very poor combination.

A classic example of a stress reaction is the fight-or-flight response that occurs when the body senses physical danger. Adrenaline, one of the body's "stress hormones," announces its presence by producing that heart-pounding sensation familiar to anyone who has experienced a good scare.

When this happens, your blood pressure begins to rise. Blood flow to the skin and the digestive system is reduced, and a greater supply is directed toward the large muscle groups. Muscle fuels—stored fats, amino acids, and quick-energy carbohydrates—enter the bloodstream. In case of injury, platelets, the blood components that help stop bleeding, increase in number. Hearing sharpens, pupils dilate to increase the field of vision, breathing deepens to provide more oxygen, perspiration increases to keep the body cool, and, finally, muscles tense in preparation for action. With all this going on, the last thing the body needs is a meal. That's why eating under stress often causes heartburn, bloating, indigestion, and nausea.

Good Nutrition Can Help

Sensible food choices can help buffer the effects of stress, for nutrients not only affect how well the body handles stress, they help determine how fast the body recovers. It's known, for example, that stress can increase the need for such nutrients as vitamin C, the B vitamins, magnesium, and zinc.

For most folks, these increased requirements can be met by a healthy diet that supplies the recommended dietary allowances (RDAs). But for individuals under severe stress, such as physical injury or surgery, there may be a need for supplements. In these cases it's best to consult a health professional, such as a trained nutritionist or a physician with nutrition savvy, for recommendations tailored to your specific needs.

During stressful periods you don't want food sitting in your stomach for long periods of time. *So avoid large meals or foods laden with fats,* such as hot dogs, cheeseburgers, french fries, and chips. Instead, stick to smaller meals containing plenty of complex carbohydrates, such as fresh vegetables, fruits, and grains. They help sustain energy, are typically high in important nutrients, and don't load you down.

Limit your intake of caffeine before periods of anticipated stress and after times that tensions have been high. Cut back on salt, particularly if you have high blood pressure. And although alcohol might be a tempting remedy for chronic stress, the potential for abuse is well known. If taken in lieu of a healthy diet, alcohol drains the body of needed nutrients and hastens one's demise.

Because the stress response brings muscle fuels to the bloodstream, *exercise* is an important part of any stress-relief formula. Any exercise routine, such as going for a brisk walk or forsaking the elevator for the stairs, can help release tensions and return you to a calmer state.

If you're at the dining-room table and stress makes an unexpected appearance, stop eating. If possible, try to excuse yourself for a brief period. If you can't get away, use the act of eating to help put the skids on your tension. First, concentrate on taking a few, very slow, deep breaths before you continue your meal. Then, as you place foods in your mouth, focus on the different tastes and the physical act of chewing and swallowing.

Danger exists for individuals under chronic stress who either have a poor diet or are at high risk for cardiovascular disease. The increased level of circulating fats from the stress response means there will be an increase in the blood cholesterol level as well. When you also consider the increased level of clot-producing blood platelets and the higher blood pressure, it's easy to see why stress is associated with a higher incidence of strokes and heart disease.

Stress can also blunt the effectiveness of the immune system, the body's protector against infection and disease. Colds, for example, are more common after periods of stress.

If the stresses in your life are unavoidable, it's especially important to start your day with a healthy breakfast. A morning meal of protein, carbohydrates, and some fat can help stabilize your blood-sugar level and make your body better equipped to handle upcoming challenges. To be sure, people under stress should learn to handle their reactions as well as their diet. But nutrition is an important tool, and food selection is one factor you can control.

Coffee: Any Grounds for Concern?

Many of us—myself included—who make a special effort to prepare healthy meals with fresh ingredients wouldn't consider starting the day without coffee. In spite of periodic warnings that the caffeine in coffee might not be healthy, we're quite willing to ignore its failings and keep the faith with our morning brew.

This loyalty is likely due to a combination of acquired taste, personal habit, and the addictive buzz the drink doles out. But how much are we drinking coffee for the taste, and how much because we dislike the way we feel when we miss our daily dose of caffeine?

To no one's surprise, caffeine stimulates the brain. Its other effects include an increase in heart rate, an increase in acid release by the stomach, quicker transport of food through the digestive system, and a relaxation of the smooth muscles such as those found in the lungs. Caffeine also is a diuretic, which means it increases the volume of urine produced by the body. Once in the body, caffeine goes just about everywhere. In a woman, this may mean it makes its way to a developing fetus or into breast milk. Because caffeine is a foreign substance, the body will start eliminating it as soon as it appears.

Caffeine's "half-life" varies. Those who break down caffeine fastest are smokers and, strangely enough, children. It takes them about three hours to eliminate half their body's caffeine. The half-life for the average nonsmoking adult is five to seven hours. For women taking birth control pills, the rate increases to thirteen hours. The half-life in pregnant women is eighteen to twenty hours, but returns to normal levels within a month after delivery. A newborn does not gain any real ability to metabolize caffeine until he or she is several days old. Any caffeine received through mothers' milk during this period has a half-life of about three to four days. These are important points to consider for pregnant and nursing women.

Caffeine has a mixed safety record. Although it's on the FDA's GRAS List (Generally Regarded As Safe), caffeine has a dark side. Over the years, caffeine has had an on-again, off-again connection with ulcers, heartburn, cardiovascular disease, fibrocystic breast disease, cancer, birth defects, and behavioral problems stemming from its stimulant quality.

Just being associated with such diseases might be enough to give coffee a bitter taste. Yet many refuse to give up coffee—or at least switch to decaf. Some explanation may lie in the fact that the evidence is inconclusive. One study reports that caffeine is a problem, only to be followed by another saying that it really isn't that bad.

What is well accepted is that the body easily becomes addicted to caffeine. Depending on the daily intake, an abrupt withdrawal of caffeine usually will lead to withdrawal symptoms ranging from a simple headache to nausea, drowsiness, depression, and reduced attention span. These tend to be short-lived, however, and most can be avoided by cutting back on caffeine gradually.

People who drink as little as two cups of coffee a day may experience these withdrawal effects. In a study published in the *New England Journal of Medicine,* half of the sixty-two coffee drinkers experienced moderate to severe headaches when they stopped drinking coffee, and about one in ten reported depression and anxiety. The symptoms were connected to the caffeine; those who discontinued coffee but received caffeine capsules did not report the same problems.

Besides withdrawal effects, though, there are no well-established problems with caffeine in moderate amounts, meaning no more than a few cups a day. That's based on the assumption that you're a healthy, nonpregnant, non-nursing adult.

The actual line between dose and overdose can begin as low as 300 milligrams a day, but this varies greatly from individual to individual (A 6-ounce cup of drip coffee contains about 150 milligrams of caffeine; a 12-ounce cola contains about 45 milligrams.) The signs that you've had too much include headaches, muscular tremors, palpitations, nervousness, irritability, and stomach distress.

I guess I will continue to drink coffee as long as I continue to enjoy it—not because I believe that it's health food, but because I believe it's not so bad if we don't overdo it. Coffee is more than a mere beverage. While its stimulant quality may certainly be valued by many, there is an entire social ritual that revolves around coffee. It includes an aroma, the holding of a warm cup, the scent of the brew, and a sense of sharing—which curiously seems to be present even if one is drinking it alone.

11. Food Allergies and Adverse Reactions

In 100 A.D. Lucretius said, "One man's meat is another man's poison." I doubt if he was referring to food allergies, but the words certainly apply. There are many different types of adverse reactions to food, though they're not all allergies.

Food Allergies

A food allergy is the immune system's reaction to a particular food. It occurs when the body's immune system believes that a normally harmless food is an invader out to cause harm. The immune system dutifully rises to the challenge and goes into battle with this supposed adversary. The fallout from the skirmish can be symptoms ranging from sneezing, runny nose, asthma, skin rashes, nausea, diarrhea, swelling, and headache, to a life-threatening drop in blood pressure.

The first step is called *sensitization*. It usually occurs when part of a food is somehow absorbed before it's completely digested. There is a greater risk of this happening during the first six months of life, before the digestive system is fully mature.

Almost immediately after it is absorbed, the food fragment runs into the immune system, the body's security police. Because this fragment is where it doesn't belong, the immune system carries out its mission to attack and eliminate all trespassers. Then, to prepare for any future encounters, the immune system sets up a long-term defense plan. It creates a special protein called an IgE antibody, and at this point the body is said to have been sensitized. If this food is ingested again, the immune system responds again, and this time the antibodies react with the food and producing allergy symptoms.

Frequent Culprits

Although people can be allergic to anything, about 90 percent of food allergies involve peanuts, eggs, milk, wheat, tree nuts, shellfish, and soy. It's thought that the particular protein structures in these foods may have a peculiar ability to slip through the intestinal wall.

At present, the only real treatment for a food allergy is avoidance. When processed foods are eaten, this means reading the ingredient lists on each food you are considering eating. If the food you're allergic to is used throughout the food supply, avoiding a reaction can be quite difficult. For example, being allergic to corn would mean also avoiding any food that contained a corn by-product, such as corn syrup, a common sweetener in processed foods.

How Is an Adverse Reaction Different?

An adverse reaction refers to any time you react to a food in an undesirable way. All allergies are adverse reactions, but not all adverse reactions are allergies. Adverse reactions are often mislabeled allergies. Two in particular—lactose intolerance and reactions to food additives—are good examples.

Lactose Intolerance

Many people report stomachaches, bloating, gas, or diarrhea after drinking milk. This is *not* necessarily a milk allergy. More likely it reflects a reduced ability to digest the carbohydrate lactose found in milk. While uncommon in children, about 70 percent of the world's population develops lactose intolerance upon entering adulthood.

One solution to lactose intolerance is to avoid all milk products. But often, people with lactose intolerance are able to consume dairy products as part of a meal containing some fat, which helps by slowing the release of the problem-causing lactose from the stomach. Many folks are also able to eat cheese because it contains lactose in smaller amounts. Yogurt is another option; the bacteria in the yogurt culture make their own enzyme that digests the lactose for you. One final solution is to treat milk with lactase drops or take lactase pills along with milk. Your supermarket dairy section may even stock one of the brands of milk that contains pre-digested lactose.

Food Additives and Preservatives, and Gluten

People sensitive to preservatives, the flavor enhancer monosodium glutamate (MSG), food coloring, and sulfites in wine or dried fruits may experience reactions resembling those of an allergy. These are not considered food allergies, however, because they don't involve the immune system. That's no consolation for those who suffer from these types of adverse reactions, because the only practical remedy is to switch to foods that don't contain these additives.

Gluten is a complex protein found in wheat, barley, rye, and oats. In wheat flour, gluten's elastic properties contribute the springiness to dough and baked goods. An acute intolerance to this protein gives rise to celiac disease, also called nontropical sprue. In a sensitive individual, the presence of gluten can disrupt the absorptive surface of the intestines. The symptoms of the intolerance, which affects about one out of every 2,000 people, varies from mild upset stomach to a more serious condition where the digestive system can no longer digest and absorb food. Medical tests can confirm if a gluten intolerance is present. The only known treatment is to avoid all food containing gluten. There are several gluten-free cookbooks and mail-order companies that supply gluten-free foods. Contact the Gluten Intolerance Group, PO Box 23053, Seattle, WA 98102-0353.

Uncovering the Culprit

Figuring out whether a food allergy or an adverse reaction exists, and then pinpointing the culprit, can be extremely difficult. Not only are the symptoms typical of common illnesses, but the same food allergy causing a runny nose in one person could cause a life-threatening reaction in another.

Conditions under which you eat the suspect food may also play a role. Stress, infection, or nutrient deficiencies, because they have an effect on the immune system, might make you susceptible to a food allergy reaction that might not under normal conditions take place. The mystery is further complicated in that some reactions can have a delayed onset of hours or even days!

If you have allergy symptoms that you believe are food-related, it's helpful to keep a food diary. By recording all your meals and then comparing this record with your allergic reactions, you may see some pattern.

Always seek qualified assistance if you or a member of your family want to investigate a possible food allergy. Physicians who are board-certified through the American College of Allergy and Immunology are recommended. Approach with caution any practitioners who feature quick-fix methods that sound too good to be true.

12. Diet Against Cancer

The National Cancer Institute estimates that nearly half of American men and more than one third of American women will develop cancer at some time in their lives. As frightening as this sounds, it's important to realize that cancer is a disease over which we have a remarkable degree of control—more than you might realize. One risk factor is coming from a family with a member that has already had cancer, but even a family history of cancer is not a legacy written in stone. You can inherit a greater risk of cancer, but whether you get cancer depends on an interaction between that risk and a number of environmental and lifestyle factors.

And even if you get cancer, the outlook is no longer as bleak as it once was. Doctors are doing a better job of identifying and treating cancers before they can become a life-threatening problem. In the last thirty years, five-year survival rates in children under age fifteen, for example, have increased from less than 30 percent to more than 70 percent.

Cancer is not one disease, but a variety of different conditions that share at least one common characteristic, namely, that cells grow in a way that's out of control. Simply put, cancer stems from a "mistake" in a cell's DNA—the inherited genetic blueprint that tells a cell what to do. Substances that alter genes fall into two categories: *mutagens,* which cause genetic changes that may or may not lead to cancer; and *carcinogens,* which alter genes in ways known to cause cancer. All carcinogens, therefore, are mutagens, but not all mutagens end up being carcinogens.

The immune system, the body's internal police force, is designed to recognize irregular cells as well as foreign substances. As a result, most aberrant cells are identified and eliminated before any harm is done. Cancer takes root either when the immune system is not up to par, or when a cell's DNA is reprogrammed in a way that confounds any attempts at control. But even then, cancer is not a sure thing; precancerous cells can survive only if conditions favor their growth.

Tobacco remains at the top of the cancer risk list, being responsible for more than a quarter of all cancer deaths in the U.S. The other major player is diet. Scientists now estimate that at least 50 percent of all cancers can be prevented by changes in diet. What we eat (or fail to eat) will either help or hurt our body's anticancer campaign.

As a rule, it's best to limit your intake of foods known to contain higher levels of mutagens or carcinogens. These include salt-cured, smoked, and nitrite-preserved foods, such as hams or sausages. Barbecued foods, particularly those having a charred crust, should also be limited, and fish from suspect waters should be avoided.

But where diet is concerned, the keys should be *variety* and *moderation.* Variety helps to broaden your nutritional horizons; moderation lessens the risk from overemphasizing any one food. In the case of diet and cancer, these have particular significance; two examples will help to illustrate this point.

A potent carcinogen named *aflatoxin* is produced by a mold that grows on peanuts. Peanut processing companies are doing an excellent job sorting out and removing any moldy peanuts *before* they get into your food. Someone, however, who eats peanut butter every day would stand a slightly greater risk of being exposed to this carcinogen than someone who eats it only occasionally. By eating a varied diet, you lessen your chances of overloading on any one carcinogen.

Likewise, food processors use *nitrites* as preservatives in cured and smoked meat products such as hot dogs, bacon, sausages, and pastrami. The nitrites are used primarily because they are effective in preventing botulism, an often-fatal food poisoning. The nitrites themselves, however, are a mixed blessing because they can form cancer-causing chemicals called nitrosamines. The risk, however, would be negligible as long as these foods were not eaten on a regular basis.

Most epidemiological studies identify a high-fat, low-fiber diet as the type most often associated with a high incidence of cancer. The American Cancer Society supports the current guideline of limiting dietary fat to no more than 30 percent of Calories. Some studies indicate, however, that even this may be too high, and recommend that fat intake be no more than 25 percent.

It may turn out that the type of fat is the key. A study in the *Journal of the National Cancer Institute* involved interviews with 820 Greek women having newly diagnosed breast cancer and 1,548 women who were cancer-free. In analyzing the women's food habits the scientists uncovered important connections between breast cancer and a healthy diet.

The strongest link was found between the intake of vegetables and fruits and a decreased risk of breast cancer. The scientists found no link between total fat consumption and the risk of the disease. This is similar to other studies that have attempted, unsuccessfully, to connect fat intake with breast cancer. A different picture emerged, however, when the fat components were looked at individually.

The scientist found a significant link between the consumption of olive oil and a *decreased* risk of the disease. No link was found between breast cancer and the consumption of butter, and none was found with seed oils. But when they examined the role of margarine—a partially hydrogenated product of these same seed oils—the scientists found that the level of intake was tied to an *increased* risk for the disease.

The is not the first time that the intake of partially hydrogenated fat has been linked to an increased risk of breast cancer. Population studies in Denmark and the Netherlands had previously found significant associations between the consumption of hydrogenated fat and the risk of breast cancer.

When eating processed foods, stick to those with low or no partially hydrogenated fat. If you consume a large amount of processed foods, start checking the ingredient list. You'll likely be shocked to see how many foods are made with partially hydrogenated oils. As most snack foods tend to be high in fat, these are the first ones to watch.

In keeping with these recommendations, the use of shortening and spreadable fats should be kept to a minimum. When using a spreadable fat, though, consider small amounts of butter or make your own "soft" spread by mixing butter with a liquid, monounsaturated oil such as canola, olive, or almond oil. If choosing a margarine, opt for a liquid or a tub margarine—one that does not list partially hydrogenated fat first or second on the list of ingredients.

Another key anticancer strategy is to increase your intake of dietary fiber. There's a large body of evidence that associates dietary fiber with a decreased incidence of colon cancer. There's also preliminary evidence that a high fiber intake may protect against breast cancer and other cancers as well.

The foundation of your diet should be whole, fresh foods. Whenever possible include those foods that contain antioxidant nutrients such as the carotenoids, vitamins A,

C, and E, selenium, and zinc. These nutrients have a proven ability to stop or suppress many of the elements known to contribute to the cancer process. These, however, are only those nutrients for which there is already a recognized role. Scientists continue to identify other important health-promoting ingredients in whole foods.

Finally, keep in mind that the body does not passively wait for cancer to develop. It has a host of defensive systems set up to prevent cancer from occurring. However, as widespread and effective as our defensive potential might be, if the anticancer guns are nutritionally unmanned, the cancer process has a better chance of gaining ground. On the other hand, although good nutrition can protect us, it cannot make us invincible. Repeated exposure to cancer risk factors such as tobacco, excess sun, or harmful chemicals is going to take its toll, regardless of what we eat.

Diet and Ovarian Cancer

Ovarian cancer is the fifth leading cause of death in women. The menacing nature of this cancer, which accounts for about 20,000 cases every year, stems from our limited understanding of its causes and the lack of practical screening methods for early detection. A study in the *Journal of the National Cancer Institute* looked at the dietary habits of 1,014 women living in Ontario, Canada; 450 of the women had been diagnosed with ovarian cancer; the remaining 564 women were selected at random. The intent of the study was to evaluate the degree to which the intake of saturated fat increased the risk of ovarian cancer.

Through the use of questionnaires, the scientists recorded the volunteers' dietary habits. They then analyzed the diets, comparing the levels of different nutrients with the presence or absence of cancer.

The data revealed that the women who developed ovarian cancer were more likely to have diets higher in saturated fat and lower in fiber from vegetables. To place these findings in a risk-reduction context, women consuming a typical high-fat, low-fiber diet can decrease their odds of getting ovarian cancer by 20 percent if they lower their saturated fat intake by 10 grams per day.

For fiber, the risk of ovarian cancer decreased an impressive 37 percent for every 10 additional grams of vegetable fiber in the diet. (Good sources of vegetable fiber include legumes, root vegetables, and leafy vegetables.)

Ovarian cancer is an atypical cancer because it has a strong hormonal component. Women with higher levels of the hormone estrogen are known to be at higher risk. The risk reduction associated with fiber could stem from its ability to tie up estrogen in the digestive tract and usher it out of the body.

Bran News About Colon Cancer

A study published in the *Journal of the National Cancer Institute* found beneficial effects from wheat bran and calcium on the risk of colon cancer. The report was the result of a nine-month study that looked at ninety-five men and women, fifty to seventy-five years of age. All had previously had polyps removed from their large intestine, or colon. Polyps are abnormal growths that develop from the tissue that lines the colon. Although most prove to be harmless, virtually every cancer of the colon or rectum had to begin as a polyp. At present it is estimated that up to 50,000 Americans die from colon cancer every year.

The subjects were randomly assigned to groups that received either a high-fiber cereal (13.5 grams of fiber per box), or a low-fiber cereal (2 grams of fiber per box), with

either a high-calcium supplement (250 mg calcium carbonate) or placebo calcium supplement (0 mg calcium carbonate). The study was "blind" in that subjects did not
know which treatment they were receiving. The subjects
were examined at three and nine months and the fecal levels of bile acids were checked.

After nine months, those receiving the high-fiber cereal
had significantly lower levels of bile acids. Similar but
less-significant results were found in those receiving the
calcium supplement. The greatest benefit was found in
those who received the high-fiber cereal together with the
calcium supplement.

Calcium can neutralize the "acid" nature of the potentially damaging bile acids, rendering them less dangerous
to have around. The fiber, in turn, keeps things moving.
The combination of the two, as demonstrated in the study,
appears to provide a one-two-punch that can significantly
reduce the risk of colon cancer.

Barbecue: A Lesson in the Risk of Grilling

Barbecuing is a popular way of preparing food because
it's convenient and it lends a unique and appealing taste.
You have to weigh this, however, against the fact that the
grilling process can create a couple of unsavory compounds in the foods we eat.

First, when you use hot coals to cook protein foods such
as meat, pork, chicken, or fish, mutagens get formed as the
food is charred. Then, during cooking, as fat drippings hit
the hot coals, the potent carcinogen *benzopyrene* is formed.
It rises in the smoke and gets carried back to the food.

Mutagens are so named because they have the ability to
cause mutations, or changes in a cell's genetic material.
The danger is not so much that a mutation occurs, it's what

the result of the changes might be. Some mutations are harmless, but others can lead to cancer and birth defects. A carcinogen, on the other hand, is a substance that has been shown to cause cancer.

This tells us what *can* occur without saying anything about the chances that it actually will. Do we have a real danger here, or is it one that can legitimately be ignored? To help answer this we need to know about the concept of *relative risk*. This is not the danger our in-laws will drop by; it's an important way of viewing one hazard in relation to another.

Statistics show that we will increase our odds of death by one in a million through any of the following actions:

- Traveling 300 miles by car.
- Eating 400 tablespoons of peanut butter.
- Rock climbing for 1.5 minutes.
- Bicycle riding for 10 minutes.
- Having one chest X-ray taken in a good hospital.
- Canoeing for 6 minutes.
- Spending 20 minutes being a man aged 60.
- Eating 100 charcoal-broiled steaks.

Bikers, taxi drivers, canoers, rock climbers, and *especially males over sixty* would feel that these risks are tolerable. Despite this, however, we cannot deny that they exist.

Take, if you will, the danger of being hit by a car as we cross the street. One does not walk against the light in heavy traffic, nor do sane people parade through the crosswalk stripes as a vehicle speeds down the street. Precautions are needed. Assuredly, the more time spent crossing the street, the greater one's hazard.

The point here is not to dismiss risk in a cavalier manner. If you char your foods, the substances will be formed. If you eat charbroiled foods, they will enter your body.

In this case, however, there are steps to take to lessen your risk.

For example, you can limit the charring and burning by keeping the foods a minimum of six inches above the coals. You can limit the carcinogen-bearing smoke by limiting basting while grilling. Another possible solution is to arrange it so that the food isn't directly over the coals.

Plan ahead, extend cooking times, and keep temperatures more moderate by controlling air flow. The lower the heat, the less smoke and charring.

If cooking chicken, leave the skin on for the grilling, then remove it before you eat. This not only removes the charred part, but it takes the saturated fat with it.

Consider precooking your foods in a conventional or microwave oven. This limits the time spent on the grill without having major effects on the flavor.

The other foods in your diet can also work for you. We have learned that fiber adds to bulk and has the potential to lessen your exposure to whatever mutagens might be present. In addition, vegetables in the crucifer family, such as broccoli, cauliflower, and brussels sprouts, contain known anticarcinogenic substances. Fruits and vegetables rich in vitamins A and C can give you the benefit of these proven cancer fighters.

And, finally, never lose sight of the big picture. In the case of barbecue, if you are concerned about your food while sitting outside in the sun unprotected by sunscreen, or are smoking, eating a fatty diet, leading an inactive lifestyle, or drinking alcohol in excess, your priorities are all wrong. These factors represent a much greater risk than the foods on the grill.

13. Guidelines for Weight Loss

There are a host of dieting options, from do-it-yourself regimens to over-the-counter diet pills and milk shakes to formal diet programs. While clever gimmicks and persuasive testimonials might lure you—and you even might succeed at dropping a few pounds—ultimate success comes down to this: Is the method a temporary fix, or does it help you keep weight off for good?

Failure at weight loss is so common that many experts say it's the likely result of any attempt to shed unwanted pounds. Studies focusing on long-term follow-up often find that only 5 to 10 percent of dieters manage to keep the weight off.

If you number among those planning to tackle a weight problem, here are a few strategies to help improve your odds for success. A key first step is understanding what you're up against, and that means thinking of dieting from the *body's* perspective.

We tend to consider a weight-loss diet to be a planned event. But it's important to realize that a diet comes as a total surprise to the body, whose many control systems cannot recognize the difference between a diet and an actual famine. Though we "know" what we are doing and we have some idea how long the diet will last, the body's defense mechanisms are not in the loop; it assumes that a scarcity of food is the new status quo, and its innate drive for survival is activated.

Similar to the way you would cut back on spending if

your salary were cut, the body shifts into economy mode. Exactly what happens depends on the severity of the diet. Actions might include a slowing of metabolism, lowering of body temperature, or other cutbacks that leave you feeling short of energy and interested in sleep.

Who Meets with Success?

Although many studies have focused on the type of diet, too little attention has been given to the personality of the dieter. Are there traits shared by people having similar weight-loss experiences? If so, can we use this information to guide people toward programs better suited to their needs?

One study conducted through Kaiser Permanente in Oakland, California, put women into three groups: relapsers, who had lost weight and then regained it; maintainers, who lost weight and kept it off, and controls, women who had always maintained a static non-obese weight. The volunteers were questioned on weight history, dieting history, childhood food experiences, meal and snacking patterns, emotion-related eating, and methods used for handling troubling situations.

Several significant differences were noted. Relapsers typically skipped breakfast and went on restrictive diets that denied them many of the foods they enjoyed. They were more likely to take appetite suppressants and participate in formal weight-loss programs, and to seek assistance from support groups, diet partners, or health professionals. Most maintainers, on the other hand, did not seek or want help. When using the same approach to weight loss, relapsers adapted their lifestyle to the program while maintainers usually tailored the program to fit their lifestyle.

During the weight-loss period, both maintainers and relapsers reported stressful events involving family, jobs, or careers. However, maintainers tended to confront and work on these issues, while relapsers often resorted to avoidance behavior such as eating, sleeping, or drinking more, or simply wishing the problem would go away. Another significant finding was that 90 percent of the maintainers, versus 34 percent of relapsers, engaged in exercise at least three times a week.

All these findings point to personality as a significant determinant for success in long-term weight reduction. But more important, they demonstrate that there's no such thing as a one-size-fits-all plan.

While most commercial ventures suggest that their programs will work for anyone, their main accomplishment may be only a short-term loss. As suggested by the Kaiser study, people who seek treatment for a weight problem should be screened and guided into one that suits their personality. Additionally, regardless of what these programs' brochures claim, one day the program ends and you will have to call the shots.

It goes without saying that everyone interested in losing weight would like to be a "maintainer." In the Kaiser study, some of the maintainers had at one time been relapsers. But to make the change, relapsers not only had to learn how to lose weight, they had to take part in a program that understood and helped support some basic changes in personal habits. As often happens with new behavior, the road is rough in the beginning. But what you learn as part of your weight-loss regimen can eventually become a part of a normal pattern. For example, no longer would you exercise to lose weight; rather exercise becomes part of a new, healthier lifestyle that you enjoy in and of itself. The key seems to be not focusing solely on the diet. Changes in lifestyle, such as increasing your level of physical activity, can help swing the balance—and this could be nothing more than a daily brisk walk.

Before you begin, take a good long look at yourself and the

other members of your family. Do you tend to gain weight without overeating? It's well established that a tendency to retain extra weight runs along family lines. Coming from a large-framed family doesn't mean you have to abandon hope of losing weight, but it can help you set realistic goals.

Next, understand that your motivation must come from within. Attempts to change your weight solely at the behest of others are usually doomed to failure. While you may drop pounds a-plenty, your chances for long-term success are only as good as your personal commitment.

Many advertised programs may tout an ability to bring about radical change, but such results are not the norm. Your best approach is a long-term strategy, where changes are subtle and lasting as opposed to drastic and short-lived.

And this gradual shift should not emphasize only reducing Calories; it must include an activity component. Exercise not only burns Calories, it checks the slowdown of the rate at which your body burns Calories—a natural side effect of dieting.

Strategies for Success

- **Meal planning.** Eat three meals a day and select definite portions before the meal. If you're still hungry after the main course, fill up on salad, vegetables, fruits, and breads. Meal composition may be equally as important as Calories. In looking at weight changes in a group of 303 women over one- and two-year periods, scientists found that those who lowered their amount of dietary fat were more successful at weight loss than those who simply decreased their Calories.
- **Drink plenty of liquids.** Adding more liquids to your diet, such as low-Calorie beverages or soups and about eight glasses of water a day, provides fullness and helps cut down on the number of Calories you eat.

- **Focus on 5-a-day.** Try to have at least five servings of fruits and vegetables every day. (A typical serving is a medium piece of fruit, 1 cup of a leafy vegetable, 1/2 cup of fruit or cooked vegetables, 1/4 cup of dried fruit, or 6 ounces of fruit or vegetable juice.)
- **Eat slowly.** The body doesn't provide instant feedback that it has had enough food. Pace your meals to a minimum of twenty to thirty minutes in length. Eating rapidly until you're stuffed usually means you've had too much. If you like to snack, have low-Calorie snacks available for those times when you're most likely to reach for a bite.
- **Keep your activity level up.** Introduce new activities, such as riding a bike or taking a walk. Set up a schedule, possibly as a commitment made with friends, in which you ride or walk together at least three times a week. Make walking and taking the stairs a part of your daily routine. Park away from the entrance to work or shops rather than hunting for the closest space.
- **Track your efforts and reward your accomplishments.** Select a way to score your progress, and set up a series of incentive rewards for reaching intermediate goals. Consider enlisting the help and participation of other family members.
- **Shift to a weekly or even a monthly weight check.** Body weight is a sum of fat, muscle, bone, and water, and does not always reflect changes in body fat. Understand that there will be periods during which your scale weight will not change despite continued adherence to your plan. As you begin to lose weight, alter or replace clothes that no longer fit. You'll immediately know if lost pounds begin to reappear.

Why Not You?

While grim success statistics might seem to justify keeping your dieting aspirations at bay, bear in mind that such results are usually based on follow-up of individuals enrolled in formal programs. And even with this, some people succeed—so why not you? With conviction and good planning, positive results can be achieved. And even if you fall short of your desired goal, the above strategies will definitely result in a healthier you.

What About Diet Pills?

There are prescription medications that can be very effective at suppressing one's urge to eat. Some are based on amphetamines, or "speed," while others may possibly act on the hunger control center in the brain.

The difficulty with diet pills is that people often regain their lost weight. One long-term study using these drugs used 120 obese individuals. The participants lost significant amounts of weight—an average of 30 pounds in eight months—and maintained the weight loss as long as three years. More importantly, however, when the volunteers stopped taking the drugs at the end of the experiment, the weight was regained in short order.

In my opinion, except for cases in which the obesity represents an immediate threat to one's health, relying on pills to lose weight does not represent a step toward any long-term solution to a weight problem. It's better to concentrate on long-term changes in eating and activity habits. While not as fast or as easy as taking a pill, such changes when accomplished will last a lifetime.

BMI: Body Mass Index

The easiest and most-often-used methods used to evaluate weight are to get on the scale, or to take a peek at the "naked truth" by spending a few moments in front of the mirror. This coupled with how we fit in our clothes is usually enough for us to get a good idea of where we stand weight-wise. The difficulty with these self-measures is that it's hard for many to be objective. This is especially true with teenagers, where aberrant self-perceptions might encourage them to think they need to weigh much less than might be in their best interest.

This being the case, it's best to rely on established standards. For a long time this meant height/weight tables, those lengthy tables arranged according to male and female, small, medium, and large frame size, with ranges of acceptable weights for each given height. These were typically put together by insurance companies from data they gathered on individuals that lived the longest.

A better measure now being used is the BMI, which stands for body mass index. It is a more accurate way of looking at weight that takes a person's height into account.

You can calculate your BMI by dividing your weight in kilograms by the square of your height in meters. This is converted to pounds and feet in the following table.

Find your height in the column on the left, then move along that row, finding the body weight closest to yours. The number at the top of that column is your BMI. For example, if you were 5'4" tall and weighed 157 pounds your BMI would be 27. If you were 6 feet tall and weighed 175 pounds your BMI would be 24.

Federal guidelines suggest that our BMI should remain below 25. For a woman, obesity (20 percent above the desirable range) begins with a BMI over 27.5 and serious obesity (40 percent above desirable weight) begins at 31.5. For a man, obesity begins with a BMI of 28.5 and serious obesity begins with a BMI above 33.

Don't get hung up on the numbers, though. Regardless of what you weigh, you need to aim for the highest level of health by eating well and remaining active.

Body Mass Index

	19	20	21	22	23	24	25	26	27	28	29	30	35	40
4'10"	91	96	100	105	110	115	119	124	129	134	138	143	167	191
4'11"	94	99	104	109	114	119	124	128	133	138	143	148	173	198
5'	97	102	107	112	118	123	128	133	138	143	148	153	179	204
5'1"	100	106	111	116	122	127	132	137	143	148	153	158	185	211
5'2"	104	109	115	120	126	131	136	142	147	153	158	164	191	218
5'3"	107	113	118	124	130	135	141	146	152	158	163	169	197	225
5'4"	110	116	122	128	134	140	145	151	157	163	169	174	204	232
5'5"	114	120	126	132	138	144	150	156	162	168	174	180	210	240
5'6"	118	124	130	136	142	148	155	161	167	173	179	186	216	247
5'7"	121	127	134	140	146	153	159	166	172	178	185	191	223	255
5'8"	125	131	138	144	151	158	164	171	177	184	190	197	230	262
5'9"	128	135	142	149	155	162	169	176	182	189	196	203	236	270
5'10"	132	139	146	153	160	167	174	181	188	195	202	207	243	278
5'11"	136	143	150	157	165	172	179	186	193	200	208	215	250	286
6'	140	147	154	162	169	177	184	191	199	206	213	221	258	294
6'1"	144	151	159	166	174	182	189	197	204	212	210	227	265	302
6'2"	148	155	163	171	179	186	194	202	210	218	225	233	272	311
6'3"	152	160	168	176	184	192	200	208	216	224	232	240	279	319
6'4"	156	164	172	180	189	197	205	213	221	230	238	246	287	328

Low-Carbohydrate Diets

Low-carbohydrate weight-loss diets can appear to be very attractive because they can deliver a significant loss of weight in a relatively short period of time. There's a catch, however, in that aside from being restrictive, quickly lost weight tends to be rapidly regained when you go off the diet. For this reason these diets are of questionable merit for most individuals.

Here's how these diets works. When you eat only protein and fat, you have effectively eliminated your body's intake of carbohydrates. This threatens the body's access to glucose. Although the fat stored in the body is our major energy reserve, the body needs small amounts of glucose to help it burn the fat correctly. Without carbohydrates (glucose), the fats are incompletely burned. The remnants of this incomplete combustion, called ketone bodies, begin to appear. As ketones can be toxic if allowed to accumulate, the body starts to eliminate them through the kidneys via the urine. The resulting condition is called ketosis, and it also occurs in uncontrolled diabetes when there's insufficient insulin to let glucose into the energy-producing (fat-burning) cells of the body. In either case, uncontrolled ketosis can upset the body's chemical balance and give rise to a dangerous condition called acidosis.

Not having enough glucose, though, means more than producing ketones. The red blood cells have an absolute requirement for glucose, and the brain requires small amounts as well. So when the diet doesn't supply any carbohydrate, the body begins to scavenge around for potential sources of glucose among its own tissues. Body protein can be used because some of the amino acids in protein can be turned into glucose. The muscles represent the body's largest reserve of protein, and like all protein tissues, they are about 80 percent water by weight. When the body begins to take apart its proteins to make glucose, all this water weight gets released and eliminated, and like magic your weight begins to drop.

The shortage of glucose has another side effect in that you won't be bursting with get-up-and-go energy. Sure, you'll be losing some weight, but it's important to realize that a large percentage of the lost weight will be body water (a by-product of the ketosis). This weight is quickly regained once one reintroduces carbohydrates. The bottom line is that a low/no-carbohydrate diet is a questionable way to lose weight. And besides, who wants to live their life without carbohydrates?

The Yo-Yo Effect

Is it better to have lost and gained than never to have lost at all? Research on so-called "yo-yo dieting" keeps popping up—and the latest evidence indicates that individuals who continually lose and then regain weight do not have a higher risk of heart disease as was once thought.

This provides some psychological relief for the estimated 40 percent of women and 25 percent of men who say they are on a diet at any given time. Your experiences are far from unique, as estimates say as many as 90 percent of those who lose end up regaining their lost weight within a few years.

The connection between weight cycling and heart disease comes from a number of studies. A population study, for example, published in the *New England Journal of Medicine* examined 3,100 male and female volunteers ranging from twenty-nine to sixty-two years of age. These people were part of the Framingham Heart Study, an ongoing monitoring of the residents of Framingham, Massachusetts, which has been in progress since 1948. The study's analysis showed a link between how much a person's weight had changed and the risk of heart disease, or death from heart disease, as well as the risk of death from all causes. While the study did not prove that the weight cycling caused these problems, media reports at the time certainly left that impression.

Newer research has taken a closer look at this phenomenon. A study in the *Archives of Internal Medicine* (AIM) found that weigh cycling did not have a negative effect on the risk of heart disease.

The AIM research involved 101 men and 101 women who responded to a newspaper advertisement seeking participants for a weight-control study. The volunteers were put on a Calorie-restricted diet and an exercise program, with or without behavioral treatment classes to help them adhere to the regimen. Aside from measuring changes in weight, the scientists periodically measured known risk factors for heart disease, such as blood pressure, blood cholesterol level, and body fat.

After thirty months, the study found that people who cycled the most—losing 20 or more pounds and then regaining it—had the same risk of heart disease as those that had never lost the weight in the first place. The scientist in the AIM study went on to suggest that weight cycling may actually do you some good. This idea was based on the concept that a temporary lowering of risk factors may be better than no lowering at all.

This conclusion was a bit of a stretch. Heart disease is a long-term process and it's unclear what effects repeated bouts of weight cycling might have. The statement is also a rather cold way of looking at what for some can be a very frustrating occurrence.

The bottom line in the study, however, was that those that reduced their risk of heart disease the most were those that succeeded in taking weight off and keeping it off.

So we remain with our ongoing dilemma. Obesity is a known health risk, but the odds for long-term success at weight loss are dismal.

If you're interested in losing weight, how, then, should you proceed? As has always been the case, if you are on a diet, or thinking of starting one, give serious thought to what you're doing and why.

Childhood Obesity

Obesity in children is reaching epidemic proportions in this country, affecting almost one out of four children, the number having doubled in the last thirty years. This means more children are setting a course toward heart disease, diabetes, hypertension, cancer, and the other chronic health problems that currently plague the adult generation.

In defense of the "they'll grow out of it" sentiment, it is

normal for children to go through periods where they carry a little extra weight. These tend to precede an impending growth spurt and are not indicative of any long-term problem. But if the weight remains on for months or years, the odds increase that the individual will remain obese. Only 14 percent of obese infants remain obese as adults, but this number rises to 40 percent for obese seven-year-olds, and 70 percent in obese preteens. What this says is that you have a right to be concerned, and the earlier the situation is confronted, the greater the chance for change.

Although the tendency toward obesity (defined as being at least 20 percent over ideal body weight) is inherited, genetics is not the sole cause. Genetics, for example, cannot explain the increases in obesity seen over the years. Other factors, such as activity patterns and food choices, are important parts of the picture.

It's also likely that television is a major influence. Not only is TV watching passive by nature, but the TV watcher becomes fair game for attention-grabbing food commercials that use hip language, hot music, and high-tech graphics. These spots are designed to sell products, not offer nutrition education.

A study in the *Journal of the American Dietetic Association* found that about 44 percent of the commercials that saturate Saturday morning television are for foods that have little to offer besides fat and Calories. The study found that McDonald's, Burger King, and Pizza Hut accounted for 11 percent of the advertisements, and there were no commercials that focused on fruits and vegetables.

It's known that the same factors are responsible for obesity in adults and children. At home, as well as school, good nutrition and the effects of obesity need to be understood and explained. If we bribe children to eat their vegetables or clean their plate, and if sweets or high-fat treats are always looked upon as a reward, foods can soon take on a distorted value. Likewise, if parents don't follow the nutritional advice they give their children, the messages quickly lose their value.

At school, the importance of good nutrition needs to be restated and reinforced. As most of our children are unable to pass a basic physical fitness test, physical education instructors need to involve all children in activities. Involvement during the school years can be a boon to children's self-confidence and keep them socially involved and physically active. Letting them languish on the sidelines can start them on the path toward withdrawal and a negative self-image.

Once again, the key is to support good food choices as well as an active lifestyle, and to do your best to serve as a good role model. Avoid, however, becoming a dining room dictator. Studies have found that overcontrolling a child's diet can inhibit the development of a child's natural ability to regulate his or her own food intake. Such overcontrolling may lead to a higher incidence of eating disorders later in life.

If you think your child has a weight problem, an important first step is to take the child for a complete physical evaluation. Health conditions such as kidney or endocrine disorders can cause weight gain. It's important to rule out medical problems before considering changes in diet. If your physician continues to dismiss your concerns, you should consider seeking medical advice elsewhere.

In the end, you should realize that whatever might be the cause of the obesity, something can usually be done. It's easier to avoid excess fat than to take it off once it becomes part of the body.

Calories: Our Body's Energy Currency

Energy is not a nutrient. It is, however, more important than any of the other nutrients we might consume. This is because our body runs on energy, and without it everything grinds to an immediate halt—just as if someone had pulled the plug on an electrical appliance. Because it is so essential, the body has become quite good at dealing with its energy—for some of us *too good*, but more on that later.

In the United States the basic unit of energy in the body is the Calorie. A Calorie is the amount of heat energy necessary to raise the temperature of one kilogram of water, one degree centigrade.

> *If you have been wondering why there is a capital C in Calorie, it is because technically, it makes a difference whether the c in calorie is capitalized or not. One (uppercase C) Calorie is equal to 1,000 (lowercase c) calories. A Calorie might even be called a kilocalorie (kilo = 1,000). Don't be too concerned about the upper or lower case C, though. In most nonscientific literature the term calorie is assumed to mean Calorie, whether the c is capitalized or not. In other countries, they have avoided the Calorie–calorie confusion by using another unit, called the joule. If you happen to run across them, one calorie equals 4.18 joules, and one Calorie (kilocalorie) equals 4.18 kilojoules.*

You may not realize this, but fats, proteins, carbohydrates, and even alcohol are complex compounds and it requires energy to make them. We, of course, eat them as food. When your body metabolizes these compounds, or breaks them apart, the energy they contain gets released and is used by your body to do work, such as contracting muscles or manufacturing other needed compounds. One gram of fat contains approximately 9 Calories and 1 gram of protein or carbohydrate contains 4 Calories. A gram of alcohol contains 7 Calories.

How Many Calories Per Day?

The amount of energy we need in a day is dependent on how much work our bodies do. It is also dependent on age, because there is a minimum energy requirement just to keep the body's "engine" running. This is referred to as the *basal metabolism* and it gets measured in Calories. Your *basal metabolic rate*—the rate at which you burn Calories—revs up from birth until age three, when it settles down and then gradually increases until young adulthood—all the time reflecting those periods during which the body does its "growing" work. After age thirty the basal metabolic rate begins a gradual slowdown. This slowdown contributes to the tendency to gain weight as we age—particularly if we continue to eat the same amount of Calories we did when we were younger—because we may not burn all the Calories we consume.

What happens to unused calories? The body is specifically designed to hold on to every Calorie it does not need. We evolved an efficient system to deal with energy and immediately convert unneeded Calories into the form we use for storage, which is fat. We use fat because it is the most concentrated form of energy. Think of it this way: If you had to carry $1,000 around with you all the time, would you want it in coins or in paper money? If you wanted to be mobile, you would opt for paper money because it is a more concentrated form of "spending energy."

Plants, which as we know are not mobile, provide an interesting contrast. The most successful plants are those that grow the fastest so that they can spread their leaves out in the sun, which is the source of their energy. In plants, therefore, we see energy stored as carbohydrate. That's how they get the most "bang" for the Calorie "buck."

In primeval times food was a premium commodity. There were alternating periods of feast and famine and there were few forms of food preservation. Those that were the most efficient in using the Calories they ate were the ones most likely to survive. Today, famines are a thing of the past and, ironically, those that are now the most efficient at dealing with energy are the ones who tend toward obesity.

How Many Calories Do You Need?
A Two-Step Calculation
(Based on Average Day's Activity)

1. Figure Your Basal Metabolic Rate (BMR):

Women: 655 + [4.36 × Weight (lbs.)] + [4.32 × Height
(inches)] − (4.7 × Age) = BMR
Men: 66 + (6.22 × Weight (lbs)] + [12.7 × Height
(inches)] − (6.8 × Age) = BMR

2. Calculate Average Total Calories Needed Per Day:

To determine the amount of total calories, multiply your
BMR by your average activity factor listed below.

Level of Activity	Examples	Activity Factor
Very Light	Normal, everyday activities such as typing, sewing, driving, cooking, playing a musical instrument, laboratory work	1.3 (men) 1.3 (women)
Light	Walking on level surface at 2.5 to 3 mph, garage work, carpentry, golf, sailing, table tennis, housecleaning	1.6 (men) 1.5 (women)
Moderate	Walking 3.5 to 4 mph, weeding and hoeing, carrying a load, cycling, skiing, dancing	1.7 (men) 1.6 (women)
Heavy	Walking with a load uphill, tree felling, heavy manual digging, basketball, soccer, football, climbing	2.1 (men) 1.9 (women)
Exceptional	Athletes training in professional or world-class events	2.4 (men) 2.2 (women)

14. Phytochemicals:
Disease Fighters in Our Foods

Scientists looking for links between diet and disease consistently find that the incidence of killer diseases such as heart disease and certain cancers goes down as the consumption of vegetables and fruits increases. Over the years the search has been on to learn what's responsible for this effect. We know about vitamins and minerals, but is there more than this? Is it something else in the foods, or just the fact that eating more vegetables and fruits leaves you with less room for other, less-healthy fare?

We are only now beginning to grasp the power of plant substances called phytochemicals (phyto=plant). At first, beta-carotene, found in many fruits and vegetables was thought to be the key player. (Beta-carotene's antioxidant effects are discussed in chapter 5.) Research then indicated that a group of substances called the dietary flavonoids might be claiming their share of the spotlight. Anticancer compounds were found in foods of the crucifer family, which include broccoli, cauliflower, Brussels sprouts, kale, bok choi, turnips, rutabaga, and cabbage. And as scientists continued to identify other health-promoting phytochemicals, we heard about ellagic acid in grapes, isoflavones in soy, and lycopene, an antioxidant compound found in tomatoes. There seems to be a new addition to the list every month. We've known which foods contribute to good health, but science is now giving us the "chapter and verse" on the precise chemicals in our plant foods that can contribute to our well-being.

It is important to realize that phytochemicals are present for the plant's benefit, not ours! These compounds usually perform important protective functions needed to assure the plant's survival. For example, while it is understood that the sun is one of the essential forces for life, the rays of the sun can have devastating effects. Similar to the way that sunlight can "bleach" colors, a continued exposure to the sun's "oxidizing" rays might destroy a plant if they didn't have the appropriate defenses. Antioxidants and other protective phytochemicals tend to be found in the fruit and leaves that are exposed to the environment. Likewise, plants that tend to have higher levels of fats and oils will usually have an antioxidant available to protect the oil. It is only when we eat these plants, that these phytochemicals can work their protective magic for us.

Current recommendations call for a minimum of five servings of fruits and vegetables a day. Most people in the United States fail to have even half this amount. The worthy five-a-day goal, however, is not that difficult to attain as one can have more than one serving at a single meal. A typical serving is a medium piece of fruit, 1 cup of a leafy vegetable, $1/2$ cup of fruit or cooked vegetables, $1/4$ cup of dried fruit, or 6 ounces of a fruit or vegetable juice. If I were to select the best first step to help improve the average diet by adding more phytochemicals, this would be it!

Food Sources and Potential Disease-Fighting Effects of the Phytochemicals

Compound	Effects Being Investigated	Food Sources
carotenoids: alpha-carotene	antioxidant	dark green and orange fruits and

Compound	Effects Being Investigated	Food Sources
beta-carotene lectein lycopene beta-cryptoxanthin		vegetables
flavonoids (Quercitin etc.)	antioxidant	fruits and vegetables, tea, and grapes (wine)
tannins catechinine	antioxidant	green tea and some berries/wine
phenolic acids	antioxidant	parsley, cabbage, carrots, cruciferous vegetables, yams
limnoids	activate enzymes that interrupt the cancer process	citrus fruits
allyl sulfides	activate enzymes that interrupt the cancer process	onions, garlic, and scallions
indoles	activate enzymes that interrupt the cancer process	cruciferous vegetables (broccoli, cauliflower, Brussels sprouts)
dithiolthiones	activate enzymes that interrupt the cancer process	cruciferous vegetables (broccoli, cauliflower, Brussels sprouts)
isothiocyanate	activate enzymes that interrupt the cancer process	cabbage, mustard greens, horseradish, radishes, turnips

Compound	Effects Being Investigated	Food Sources
protease inhibitor	inhibits growth of cancer cells by suppressing key enzyme	soybeans
lignans	phytoestrogen: blocks estrogen activity, helping to reduce the risk of breast and ovarian cancer	flaxseed
isoflavones: genestein diadzein, glycetein	phytoestrogens (decrease risk of breast and ovarian cancer); helps decrease risk of heart disease	soybeans and soy products
fiber	binds bile acids, dilutes and reduces contact time with any potential carcinogens	whole grains, vegetalbes, and fruit
ellagic acid	helps eliminate carcinogens	strawberries, raspberries, blueberries, grapes (wine)
sulforaphane	protects against cancer	cruciferous vegetables (broccoli, cauliflower, and Brussels sprouts)
resveratrol	antioxidant, protects agains cancer	grapes, wine, peanuts

Compound	Effects Being Investigated	Food Sources
allium compounds	help lower blood pressure and blood cholesterol; possible immune-system-enhancing ability	garlic and onions
glycyrrhizin	anticancer effects	licorice root
luetin zeanthin	help prevent age-related macular degeneration	spinach and other dark green leafy vegetables
capsaicin	potential effect against ulcer-causing bacteria; may be able to neutralize carcinogenic effect of nitrosamines	peppers

Flavonoids Research

Evidence about phytochemicals comes from a crosscultural population study published in the *Archives of Internal Medicine* (AIM). The study examined dietary and health information from groups in seven countries. The data collection, begun in 1960, was a part of an ongoing examination that stretched over twenty-five years.

A total of 12,763 men, forty to fifty-nine years of age, participated in what became known as the Seven Country Study. Initiated by Dr. Ancel Keys of the University of Minnesota, information from this study has already improved our understanding of the relationship between diet and health. Reports about the role of olive oil (monounsaturated fat) and the healthfulness of the Mediterranean diet are one of its more recent outcomes.

The subject of this particular study was the flavonoids, a family of antioxidant compounds found in varying degrees in vegetables, fruits, fruit juices, tea and red wine; the highest concentrations were found in onions, kale, broccoli, endive, French beans, celery, and cranberries. These compounds attracted attention when research demonstrated how they could have potent health benefits. The scientists in the AIM study decided to examine the effects long-term flavonoid intake might have on the incidence of heart disease and cancer.

In examining the volunteers' diets and their (eventual) cause of death, the scientists found that as the intake of dietary flavonoids went up, the risk of death from heart disease was significantly decreased. No link, however, was found between flavonoid consumption and the incidence of cancer.

The study also found, not surprisingly, that heart disease increased with the incidence of smoking and the level of dietary fat. The beneficial effect of the flavonoids, however, was independent from the effects of smoking or the level of dietary fat. And, in a statement of their potential importance as health promoters, the flavonoid's beneficial effect on heart disease was greater than that seen for beta-carotene, vitamin E, or vitamin C.

The impact of this research is to highlight that what you eat is as important as what you don't. Reducing the level of fat in the diet may not be as important as eating the foods that provide the variety of nutrients your body needs to stay in good health. In addition, it's not realistic to think that supplements can capture all the goodness that healthy foods have to offer.

Because flavonoids are present in red wine, the AIM findings lend support to the "French paradox" argument that red wine consumption contributes to the relatively low rate of mortality from heart disease in red wine drinkers. Flavonoids are also found in Japanese-style green teas and they likely contribute, along with a low-fat diet, to the low rates of heart disease seen in the Japanese.

Healthful Benefits from Soy

A study in the *New England Journal of Medicine* reported on the effect of soy proteins on lowering the level of cholesterol and fats in our blood. Such findings may bring about a craze for soy-protein-spiked processed foods such as happened with oat bran, but hopefully this won't be the case. While the study touts soy protein, it may be other compounds in soybeans that are actually behind the bulk of the benefits.

The NEJM study involved "meta analysis"—a powerful statistical technique that brings together a number of studies that attempt to answer a similar question. The thirty-eight individual studies that were a part of the soy research relied on more than 730 research volunteers. The soy protein intakes in those studies ranged from 17 to 124 grams per day, with 47 grams per day as the average. In all of them, the volunteers ate soy in place of other proteins in the diet.

The analysis found that volunteers consuming soy protein experienced a drop in their blood cholesterol level of about 23 milligrams per deciliter, or about 9 percent. Those with the highest initial blood cholesterol levels benefitted the most.

The findings were particularly noteworthy in that the LDL, or least desirable cholesterol, dropped, while the HDL, or highly desirable cholesterol, was unchanged. The consumption of soy protein was also associated with a significant decrease in blood triglycerides.

These are very encouraging results for those looking for ways to tame a stubborn blood lipid problem.

The soybean has a fascinating past. Cultivated in China since the eleventh century B.C., it was considered one of the five sacred grains necessary for life. The soybean's obscure introduction to the United States came in 1804, when the beans were used as an inexpensive ballast on a clipper ship en route from China. Upon arrival, the soybeans were discarded; some, apparently, found their way to tillable soil.

Initially, soybeans were used for soy sauce, but during the Civil War the soybean found a new niche as a beverage when it was roasted in place of then-scarce coffee beans. During the late 1800s the soybean began being used as a feed crop for cattle. In the 1900s, initially through the work of agricultural scientists such as George Washington Carver, more palatable varieties were brought over from China and soybeans made the transition from forage to food.

Soybeans are unique among normally low-fat legumes in that they are approximately 40 percent oil by weight. During processing, the beans first have their oil extracted and the remaining soy mash is used as a high-protein feed for livestock.

So, despite its roots as one of the main foods in the low-fat, low-meat Asian cuisine, the soybean has found a great home in America's high-fat, meat-centered way of eating. Today, soybeans are this country's second leading cash crop, with more soybeans being grown in the U.S. than anywhere else. This latest information on the apparent healthfulness of soy protein may provide a new boon to the use of soy-based foods in the diet.

What's of particular interest, though, is that while the NEJM study focused on the beneficial effects of soy proteins, researchers don't yet know how the soy "protein" is able to accomplish this feat. There may, in fact, be other compounds in soybeans that are responsible. For example, soybeans contain compounds called *isoflavones*, which are plant chemicals unique to soybeans. These compounds have antioxidant abilities that may be playing a direct role in soy's beneficial effects.

One soy isoflavone, named genestein, even has some of the beneficial properties of the anti-estrogen drug tamoxifen used to combat breast cancer. This factor may be playing a role in the lower incidence of breast cancer seen among populations eating soy-based diets.

It was noted in both the NEJM study and an accompanying editorial that the plant compounds, such as the isoflavones, may be behind soy's cholesterol-lowering effect. Although soy protein was the focus of the study, not all soy protein preparations contain isoflavones. If, for example, a soy protein is manufactured with an alcohol-based solvent, the beneficial soy isoflavones will not be present. Is the key factor the soy protein? The isoflavones? Or, does the effect need both?

In the end, the message from the NEJM study should not be to encourage a new generation of soy-protein muffins, cookies, and doughnuts. It should be to encourage us to take a closer look at soy as a healthful whole food that deserves a place in our diet.

The Tasteful Wonders of Garlic

Garlic, a member of the lily family and a relative of the onion and scallion, continues to show its mettle beyond the widely respected ability to cure a bland meal. Throughout history, garlic has been touted for its curative properties. Ancient Greek and Egyptian writings mention garlic as an effective remedy against a variety of ailments—the ancient Egyptians using garlic on wounds and infections and to fight off intestinal parasites. In World Wars I and II, the British, German, and Russian governments put garlic extracts on bandages to help disinfect wounds. It has only been in recent years, however, that we have begun to understand the science behind the potential health applications of this herb.

Garlic has been credited with combating heart disease, stimulating the immune system, attacking bacteria, viruses, and funguses, and increasing the body's ability to resist cancer-causing agents.

The key to garlic's seemingly magical array of abilities is a phytochemical named *allicin*. But as with all phytochemicals, it's not there just for us. The garlic plant uses its allicin to protect itself from damage by insects, bacteria, and fungi. Allicin is a highly reactive compound that can be toxic in large doses and is believed to be responsible for the stinging-mouth sensation often experienced when eating raw garlic. Proteins in the saliva usually react with the allicin and render it benign, but some report stomach distress when consuming raw garlic. In one experiment, volunteers consuming doses of garlic juice on an empty stomach reported burning of the mouth, esophagus, and stomach, lightheadedness, nausea, and sweating.

What's wonderful about garlic, though, is not the allicin itself, but the fact that it breaks down into a host of powerful compounds that are a boon to health. Some of these breakdown compounds become antioxidants, others serve as anticlotting agents and detoxifiers. When garlic is cooked in oil, the allicin helps to form compounds that are patented for anti-asthma activity.

A study in the journal *Lipids* described how a garlic supplement decreased the oxidation of the blood's LDLs, the cholesterol-carrying lipoproteins associated with the risk of heart disease. LDL oxidation is believed to be one of the first steps along the road to heart disease.

Another study, in the *American Journal of Medicine,* found a significant decrease in blood cholesterol in healthy adult males after a twelve-week treatment with a standardized garlic powder. The volunteers in the study began with cholesterol levels above 220 mg/dL.

As an example of how else this pungent herb might help out, researchers at West Virginia University reported in the journal *Cancer* that mice fed a garlic extract showed a slower rate of tumor growth after being injected with cancer cells than similar mice that received no garlic. This anticancer effect may be due to garlic's ability to help activate the mouse's immune system.

Although garlic's health benefits are impressive, not all foods are improved by its unique flavor. In addition, many people do not appreciate the telltale odor that frequently emanates from an eater of garlic. The characteristic odor is created as the components of garlic are disbursed throughout the body. When they travel to the lungs, these compounds give rise to "garlic breath," and when they reach the skin, the olfactory offender becomes noticeable in perspiration. This explains why brushing one's teeth or even taking breath mints does little to suppress garlic odor.

Garlic Supplements

If you're interested in garlic but either it disagrees with you or you simply don't like the taste, there is a wide assortment of garlic supplements available in health food stores. The capsules, which often contain garlic oil extract, do not prevent odor; all they do is delay its presence until the garlic goes through the body. There are supplements, however, that are based on a deodorized, aged garlic extract, and other pills that contain standardized amounts of allicin, all of which appear to offer similar health benefits as whole-clove garlic without the odor.

Should these findings convince you to add more garlic to your diet with supplements? Unfortunately, there's no guidance about how much is needed to achieve positive health effects. In addition, there's little information on possible side effects from long-term garlic supplementation. With the mounting evidence of its health-promoting qualities, though, you should take steps to use the whole herb in your cooking. Food remains the best and unquestionably the most "tasteful" way to add garlic to your diet.

15. Alcohol and the Mediterranean Connection

In an affront to America's growing low-fat consciousness, the French diet has stormed our shores. In the print and electronic media, the French style of eating has been touted for its health benefits—this despite the fact that the diet is often seen floating in fat and is typically awash in a daily intake of red wine. The message of the campaign was clear: The French diet can provide a pleasant passport around the debacle of heart disease.

A ten-year study revealed that people in the Gascony region of southwest France live long lives and suffer relatively few deaths from heart attack—even though their diet is higher in fat than any other in the industrialized world. What is it about their cuisine that lets the French "break the rules" and still reap an apparent health advantage?

Aside from their abiding respect for and love of good food, what is often mentioned is the French habit of having wine with meals. Over the years, many studies have revealed how a moderate intake of alcohol is associated with a decrease in the risk of heart disease.

Scientific research has attested to an ability of alcohol—whether from red wine or any other source—to raise the HDL component of the blood. (The HDLs help shuttle cholesterol out of the body.) This protective effect, however, is only present with moderate intake of alcohol—defined as one to two drinks per day. (A drink is defined as a 4-ounce glass of wine, 12-ounce glass of beer, or 1-ounce shot of hard liquor in a mixed drink.)

A two-year study in the British journal *Lancet* that looked at the drinking habits of 44,000 men found there was a 25 to 40 percent lower incidence of heart disease in those with a moderate intake of alcohol. Another study, in the *British Medical Journal,* linked a moderate alcohol consumption with a similar 40 percent reduction in deaths from heart disease in men and women living in New Zealand.

An article in the *Journal of the American Medical Association* (JAMA) said that one possible mechanism behind alcohol's effect was its ability to increase the level of a substance called the t-PA antigen. This substance helps to unclog blood clots that might otherwise develop into heart-disease-causing blockages.

While positive effects have been found using different alcoholic beverages, studies in *Lancet* and in the *Journal of Applied Cardiology* have suggested that red wine may indeed contain additional components that can reduce the risk of heart disease. The difficulty, however, is knowing whether a moderate intake of any vintage of any red wine will give you enough of an effective "dose" of these beneficial substances.

The idea of moderation is an important one. Most of the nutrients we eat are absorbed after they've been broken down, or "digested," into smaller parts. But alcohol is one of the few compounds that can be absorbed directly through the lining of the stomach. This means that we tend to feel alcohol's effects sooner—especially if it's consumed on an empty stomach. The body has definite tolerances for alcohol intake. The liver is the organ that metabolizes (breaks down) alcohol, and it seems to be able to handle about one drink an hour. When the body takes in alcohol at a more rapid rate, the alcohol ends up waiting in queue to be metabolized. The holding area, it turns out, is our bloodstream, and as the concentration of blood alcohol increases, we begin to experience intoxication and alcohol's other negative effects.

Tolerance to alcohol is said to be weight-related; the larger you are, the more you can tolerate. This is not so much because those of greater size metabolize the alcohol faster, but more due to the fact that the bigger the body, the greater the volume of blood, which effectively gives you a larger holding area to dilute the alcohol and keep blood alcohol concentrations from rising as fast.

The JAMA study was accompanied by an editorial that stated if the entire U.S. population stopped drinking all forms of alcohol there would be an additional 81,000 deaths per year from heart disease. This number was placed in perspective, though, when the article also stated that there are approximately 100,000 people who die each year from alcohol-related causes.

The point was not to make a case for prohibition, but to emphasize that alcohol should never be looked upon as preventative medicine. It's better to rely on a healthy diet and a more active lifestyle. For those that take care of themselves, though, it's good to know that a moderate intake of alcohol can provide additional health benefits.

Alcohol is not the only aspect of the "French approach" that deserves our attention. In addition to having wine with their meals, the French typically eat fresh fruits, vegetables, and breads purchased on a daily basis. They spurn shortening and vegetable oils in favor of butter. And their dairy intake has twice as much cheese and skim milk and half as much whole milk and cream as typically eaten in this country.

The "Mediterranean diet," eaten in neighboring Italy and Greece, also celebrates eating while managing to marry high-fat food with a relatively low incidence of heart disease. In Italy and Greece, the diet is based more on olive oil than butter, but it shares the French focus on fresh foods and consumption of red wine with meals.

What these Mediterranean examples demonstrate is that there are many ways to approach a healthy diet. A myopic view—such as the American "low-fat is where it's at" approach—is not the only answer. Common threads among Mediterranean countries are the emphasis on freshness, a relaxed attitude, and a celebration of good food. To top it all off, these foods taste great! Now there's something we can all take to heart.

16. The Latest Shake on Salt

A salt shaker is usually nearby whenever food is served; next to sugar, we add more salt to our food than any other condiment. There is a widely held belief that too much salt will lead to high blood pressure in everyone. It turns out, however, that the connection between salt and high blood pressure may be true for only a minority of individuals. Nevertheless, there are good reasons for all of us to moderate our use of salt.

Dietary salt, which usually refers to table salt, is a chemical compound called sodium chloride. Both sodium and chloride are essential for life. *Our health, however, can be maintained with as little as $1/10$ of a teaspoon (600 milligrams) of salt per day.* By contrast, the American's average daily intake is ten to thirty-five times that amount.

Where does all that salt in our diet come from? It turns out that 10 percent is naturally present in food, 15 percent is added during cooking and at the table, and a whopping 75 percent comes from processed foods.

Why is there so much salt in processed foods? Food manufacturers find salt attractive for several reasons. Besides its role as a flavor enhancer, salt retards the growth of a variety of microorganisms. In fact, in the days before refrigeration, salting was the only practical way to keep meats and fish from spoiling.

Salt also plays a role in food texture. Processed meats

such as bologna, frankfurters, and luncheon meats contain high levels of salt because it helps form and maintain the gel-like consistency. Salt is also abundant in tomato-based products, such as spaghetti and pizza sauce and tomato juice, and it is used widely in cheese and prepared soups.

In the body, the salt/water balance must be kept within fixed limits for nerve impulses and muscle contractions to take place. Because of this, our body carefully regulates the amount of salt in its fluids and tissues.

If we ingest too much salt, the body immediately attempts to water down the excess salt, a step that's required before it can be eliminated through the kidneys. To do this, water gets pulled from inside our tissues into the bloodstream. This triggers a sense of thirst to provide more needed water. The kidneys have a limit of how much salt they can eliminate in a fixed quantity of water. Between the control of thirst and the function of the kidneys, the concentration of salt in the body varies by no more than 1 percent.

Is Salt at Fault?

Perhaps the main concern about excess salt is due to its association with high blood pressure, or hypertension. High blood pressure currently affects about 50 million Americans. It's called the silent killer because there are no warning signs until problems such as heart disease, stroke, or kidney disease have already developed. The only reliable way to find out whether you have hypertension is to have your blood pressure checked.

The connection between salt and hypertension was suggested after several population studies compared salt intake with blood pressure. Scientists found that hypertension was rare in societies eating a low-salt diet, and more common in societies, such as ours, that consume a high-salt diet. This information, together with several animal studies, led to a public health policy to lower the salt in our diet.

There is some logic to this association. After all, it was known that the body responded to a high salt intake by diluting the salt and thereby increasing the volume of fluid in the blood. Perhaps this increased blood volume was the cause of the higher blood pressure observed in the studies.

Many scientists, however, disagreed with the need for salt restriction, and the debate has gone back and forth over the years. In some cases, the population groups that had a low salt intake and a low incidence of high blood pressure also had active lifestyles and ate a vegetarian diet. In addition, further studies have found that other factors may be more effective than salt at controlling blood pressure. For example, high blood pressure usually takes a nosedive whenever excess weight or alcohol consumption is reduced.

One review article in the *American Journal of Hypertension* concluded, "There is no justification for the recommendation that salt intake be restricted in the general population to avert blood pressure rise."

Two other prestigious medical journals have also entered the salt–blood pressure debate. In one corner is the *British Medical Journal* and its report of a solid relationship between dietary salt intake and high blood pressure. Their conclusion was that everyone needs to reduce their intake of salt, this especially being the case for those that already have high blood pressure.

In the other corner is the *Journal of the American Medical Association,* which reported that some individuals, such as seniors and those who already have high blood pressure, might be helped by salt restriction, but that current data do not support salt restriction as a general public policy.

What Are We to Conclude?

Unfortunately, science has not yet come up with a way to predict who gets hypertension. At present it's known that there is a strong genetic component and that African-Americans are more likely to develop high blood pressure than European-Americans. Therefore, the key is to routinely have your blood pressure checked, particularly if you are black, but also if you are obese, have a high alcohol consumption, or tend to be inactive, as these are also risk factors for high blood pressure.

Incidentally, it's been reported that blood pressure varies throughout the day. There's even a condition called "white coat hypertension," in which blood pressure tends to rise in the presence of a health professional. Because the likelihood of a false positive (or negative) is greatest with only one measurement, it's considered best to rely on multiple measurements to confirm any diagnosis of high blood pressure.

When people with hypertension are given a low-salt diet, there are those that do indeed experience a significant decrease in blood pressure. These "salt-sensitive" hypertensives, though, are only a minority, numbering about 25 to 40 percent of those with hypertension. Salt restriction is key for these individuals. Another group that appears to benefit from salt restriction are older individuals with hypertension.

If you are at high risk, or are uncertain about your blood pressure, keep your use of salt to a minimum. Avoid reaching for the salt before you taste your food. Saltiness is one of our basic tastes, and salt can help bring out the flavor in food. The key, however, is to enjoy the natural flavor of food, not that which sits in the salt shaker.

Where Salt Hides Out

The dietary guidelines of the Food and Nutrition Board state that you should limit your sodium intake to no more than 2,400 milligrams per day. Here are some common "salty" foods along with the level of sodium they contain.

2 slices bacon	202 mg
1/2 cup cheddar cheese	350 mg
4 oz. potato chips	532 mg
1 hot dog (without bun)	638 mg
1/2 cup sauerkraut	780 mg
1 cup tomato juice	882 mg
1 medium dill pickle	928 mg
1/2 cup grated Parmesan cheese	931 mg
1 cup dry-roasted salted peanuts	986 mg
1 cup refried beans (canned)	1,073 mg
1 cup chicken noodle soup (canned)	1,106 mg
1 cup spaghetti sauce (canned)	1,236 mg
1 cup potato salad	1,323 mg
1 tsp. salt	2,300 mg

17. The Hidden Costs of Pesticide Use

In terms of variety and abundance of food, Americans number among the best fed in the world. As we go from season to season, it behooves us to consider how this lofty status comes with a tremendous price tag in natural and human resources.

U.S. agriculture uses almost 45 billion pounds of synthetic fertilizers and 845 million pounds of pesticides each year. These are manufactured primarily from petroleum, translating to a hefty 140 gallons of petroleum per acre for a major cash crop such as corn. This helps to explain why farming uses more oil than any other single industry.

Additionally, while public concern about pesticides typically focuses on potential dangers from eating the food, what about the workers who apply these often cancer-causing chemicals? And what of our environment, which becomes the final resting place for all chemicals?

The U.S. Environmental Protection Agency has found pesticides in the groundwater of over thirty states. Fertilizers also find their way into the water supply. In some areas so much nitrogen has been applied to the soil that runoff has made the groundwater unsafe for children to drink.

America's obsession with perfect-looking produce is one of the key factors behind the continued demand for pesticides. The National Academy of Sciences, in a report titled "Alternative Agriculture," detailed how the food industry encourages the use of pesticides solely to maintain high cosmetic standards. Separate surveys conducted on citrus fruits by Public Voice and the American Farm Bureau Federation found that, in some cases, over half the pesticides used are for purely cosmetic reasons, such as to prevent minor external blemishes that had nothing to do with the taste or wholesomeness of the fruit.

Many health experts place the hazards from pesticides well behind other dangers in our food supply, such as bacterial contamination and naturally occurring toxins. They say that the major risks in our food supply are placed there by nature, not technology.

However, numerous unanswered questions remain. For example, there is no practical way of measuring how, or if, an amount of residue deemed safe today might affect your health down the road. We also have no way of judging the effects of residues in combination with each other, or what happens when pesticide exposure occurs in conjunction with other health problems. That may be why, despite assurances, survey after survey reveals that American consumers continue to be wary.

There are excellent alternatives to the continued use of pesticides. One involves organic agriculture. Organically grown crops, which generally cost more to produce than most conventional foods, are raised without synthetic chemicals, such as pesticides, fertilizers, animal feed additives, or growth regulators.

Consider the contrasting ways these two approaches would deal with insect pests, a common problem faced by growers. The conventional approach would be to kill the insects by spraying chemical pesticides on the crop. By contrast, the organic approach would be to introduce a harmless insect, such as a ladybug or a lacewing, that's a natural predator to the bothersome bug. In both cases the crop would be saved, but with organics there would be no dangerous chemicals or potential residues involved in the process.

An important alternative is called integrated pest management (IPM), a compromise between conventional and organic agriculture. This approach makes use of nonchemical techniques whenever possible; however, synthetic chemicals remain a part of the farmer's arsenal that can be called upon if the situation demands it.

Opponents of organic methods argue that without chemical pesticides American farmers could no longer feed the nation, and the cost of food would skyrocket. Such claims, however, do not appear to be accurate. In a three-volume publication on pest management in agriculture, a Cornell researcher reviewed crop yields and pesticide use on hundreds of farms. He reported that farmers could cut pesticide use by as much as half with no impact on crop yields and less than a 1-percent increase in prices.

There's little question that it's better to eat conventionally grown produce than not to eat fruits and vegetables at all. Our produce market is not a hazardous place where we need fear every bite. Yet this does not justify blind support for the use of unnecessary synthetic pesticides. We should eat as though our life depended on it. And at the same time, we need to constantly be aware of the environmental impact of our food choices.

Waxes on Our Produce

Produce growers apply waxes to their fruits and vegetables to retain moisture, retard flavor loss, and enhance appearance. Petrolatum, paraffin, and carnauba are different types of waxes. Petrolatum and paraffin are petroleum (oil) by-products. Carnauba, which comes from the wax palm of Brazil, is also used in car wax. Shellac, another commonly used wax, comes from an Asian insect and is also used on candies, jewelry, and floor waxes.

Waxes are applied to a wide variety of produce, includ-

**Some Commonsense Steps to
Help Reduce Pesticide Risks**

- Wash your vegetables.
- Peel the produce whenever there's a wax coating.
- Buy produce grown locally or regionally.
- Eat fruits and vegetables in season. Those grown in other countries are not necessarily held up to the same level of scrutiny.
- Shop at farmers' markets whenever possible.
- Eat a variety of foods.
- Buy certified organic fruits and vegetables or those produced on a farm that uses IPM.
- If organically grown or IPM products are not available, speak with the produce manager of your store to see if they can be carried.

ing tomatoes, apples, bell peppers, avocados, cucumbers, sweet potatoes, all citrus fruits, peaches, pumpkins, eggplants, squash, and nuts in hard shells. The waxes are not considered harmful and are only used in small amounts. The Center for Produce Quality estimates that one pound of wax will cover 160,000 pieces of fruit or vegetables.

One potential cause for concern with waxes stems from the possible presence of pesticide and fumigant residues on the surface of the produce before the wax is applied. In some cases, the pesticide or fumigant is mixed with the wax (or the wax is applied after the treatment). When a wax is present, these chemicals cannot be washed off. The health risk posed by the presence of such wax-bound pesticides or fumigant residues should be minimal if the chemicals are applied properly. And, of course, it's only an issue for produce in which the skin is consumed.

Although you can try scrubbing these waxes off, it takes more than water to do the trick. A mild detergent, or products that claim to clean the wax off produce (available at natural food stores), may be helpful. Without these, the only real way to "de-wax" the product is to take off the peel.

There is an FDA regulation, albeit rarely followed, that requires stores to indicate which produce is waxed. The FDA is expected to include a new set of guidelines for the labeling of waxed produce as part of the new food-labeling initiatives.

Both conventional and organic growers make use of waxes. Organic growers' waxes come from natural sources and do not contain any synthetic pesticides or fungicides. The presence of waxes is yet another reason why it's best to consume a variety of fruits and vegetables rather than always sticking to one particular fruit.

PART III

The A to Z of Processed Foods

18. Food Labeling:
Why All the Fuss?

The history of the labeling and marketing of food has paralleled advancements in nutrition science. As more people became interested in the connection between diet and health, food companies began using labels and advertisements to make and market "healthful" products.

The key event occurred in 1984, when Kellogg's advertised that its All-Bran cereal was useful in the prevention of cancer. The Food and Drug Administration (FDA) had not previously allowed such claims, but Kellogg's ads had received the endorsement of the National Cancer Institute, another government organization.

The food industry waited to see whether the FDA would order Kellogg's to change its ads, but as time passed it became obvious that nothing was going to happen. Other companies followed Kellogg's lead and a flood of health claims and messages worked their way into the marketplace—each outdoing the other in proclaiming the healthfulness of their product. The situation continued to deteriorate until March 1990, when Secretary of Health and Human Services Dr. Louis Sullivan described the food label as a "Tower of Babel" in desperate need of reform. Later that year, Congress enacted the Nutrition Labeling and Education Act, which ordered the FDA to overhaul the food label.

After gathering input from a series of focus groups held around the country, the FDA came up with a new format and standardized label language that had to appear on all packaged foods by May 8, 1994.

Just the Facts

Today's food label is identifiable by the words *Nutrition Facts*. The actual type of nutrition label used depends on the size of the package. For example, no label is required for products having less than twelve square inches of available label space, but such products must list a telephone number or address for consumers to call or write for nutrition information. Small businesses are also exempt; a small business is defined as one with fewer than 100 employees that produces fewer than 100,000 units, or one with an annual gross sales of less than $500,000, or with annual gross sales of food to consumers of less than $50,000.

The first item on the label, the serving size now more accurately reflects amounts that people eat and it is standardized between different brands. (No more 1 1/3 servings in a drink box!) An ingredient list is required for all packaged foods. On this list will be all the components present in the food, listed in order of prevalence. The ingredient list appears at the end of the nutrition label.

The main part of the new label is a table comparing the amount of nutrients in one serving with the total fat, carbohydrate, fiber, protein, vitamins, and minerals that should be present in an average daily diet. It's all based on a dietary standard called the Daily Value (DV). The DVs are a one-size-fits-all allowance that are used as a reference for food labeling. They are based on an updated and expanded version of the U.S. Recommended Daily Allowances, or U.S.RDA, for vitamins, minerals, and protein that has been used on packaged foods since 1973. The Daily Value is not the same as the RDA, or recommended

Nutrition Facts

Serving Size 1/2 cup (114g)
Servings Per Container 4

Amount Per Serving

Calories 260   Calories from Fat 120

	% Daily Value*
Total Fat 13g	**20%**
Saturated Fat 5g	**25%**
Cholesterol 30mg	**10%**
Sodium 660mg	**28%**
Total Carbohydrate 31g	**11%**
Dietary Fiber 0g	**0%**
Sugars 5g	
Protein 5g	

Vitamin A 4%	•	Vitamin C 2%	
Calcium 15%	•	Iron 4%	

* Percent Daily Values are based on a 2,000 calorie diet. Your daily values may be higher or lower depending on your calorie needs:

		Calories:	2,000	2,500
Total Fat	Less than		65g	80g
Sat Fat	Less than		20g	25g
Cholesterol	Less than		300mg	300mg
Sodium	Less than		2,400mg	2,400mg
Total Carbohydrate			300g	375g
Dietary Fiber			25g	30g

Calories per gram:
Fat 9 • Carbohydrate 4 • Protein 4

dietary allowance, which is a set of nutrition standards that is tailored for men, women, and children in different age groups. The RDA, unlike the Daily Value, is periodically updated.

On the label there are Daily Values for fat, saturated fat, carbohydrate, fiber, and protein that are based on the number of Calories you eat during the day, while DVs for cholesterol, sodium, and potassium are fixed amounts.

In the table of Daily Values on the label the percent DVs are based on a 2,000-Calorie diet with 10 percent of the day's Calories coming from protein, 60 percent from carbohydrates, and 30 percent from fat (no more than one-third of which is saturated fat).

A full-size label also lists at the bottom the amounts in grams of total fat, saturated fat, cholesterol, sodium, total carbohydrate, and fiber that should be present in an average 2,000-Calorie and 2,500-Calorie diet, and a notation about the amount of Calories per gram of fat, carbohydrate, and protein. The purpose of these numbers is to let you see how one serving of the food fits into your daily diet.

When reading this information, keep in mind that a 2,000-Calorie diet may be excessive for smaller women and children, and a 2,500-Calorie diet would provide insufficient Calories for larger individuals and those that are physically active.

Calories from fat are prominently displayed alongside the total Calories per serving. You can calculate the percent of Calories from fat by dividing the Calories from fat by the total Calories and then multiplying by 100.

The vitamins and minerals required on the label are vitamins A and C and calcium, but manufacturers may include others. If a serving contains less than 2 percent of a required nutrient(s), the manufacturer can state this on the label and not have to list that nutrient(s) in table format. A food, such as coffee, which doesn't supply any nutrients, does not need to have a nutritional label.

The Missing Fat

As we have seen, of all the fats in foods, the mono-unsaturated fatty acids, such as those found in olive and canola oil, are the type that should be the focus of the diet. It may come as a surprise therefore to learn that the "heart-unhealthful" trans fatty acids (TFAs) found in partially hy-drogenated fats are also monounsaturated.

Before the Nutrition Labeling and Education Act of 1990, TFAs were included along with the other monounsaturated fats for labeling purposes. As evidence mounted against TFAs, it became obvious to many that this practice should be changed. The design of the new labels, however, was already under way. In a confusing eleventh-hour decision, the Food and Drug Administration decided that TFAs would be included in the total fat per serving, but they would not be counted as monounsaturated fats.

This means that on some labels the numbers don't add up. For example, the label for a cookie lists 7 grams of fat per four-cookie serving. The label then goes on to list the separate components of fat:

Saturated Fat . . . . 1 gram
Polyunsaturated Fat . . . . 0 grams
Monounsaturated Fat . . . . 2.5 grams

Total Fat . . . . 7 grams ???

Fat can only be saturated, monounsaturated, or poly-unsaturated, so you would think that these numbers would add up to the total. It's obvious that 1 gram + 0 grams + 2.5 grams does not equal the 7 grams of fat per serving. The unaccounted for 3.5 grams of fat per serving are the TFAs.

This won't work for all products, however. While all labels have to list both total fat and saturated fat, a complete

breakdown is only required if the product makes a claim
about saturated fat or cholesterol.

There is no doubt that the consumer would be much better served if the amount of TFAs per serving were required
to be listed on the label.

Confusing Sugar

The terms *sugar* and *carbohydrate* are often used interchangeably, and this leads to confusion when interpreting
food labels. As explained in chapter 3, technically, all sugars are carbohydrates, and carbohydrates can be referred to
as sugars. On the food label, these words have more precise meanings. It helps to understand that while all carbohydrates are made up of single-sugar building blocks, the
common sugar compounds can be made up of either one
single sugar by itself or two single sugars attached to each
other, referred to as double sugars. For the purposes of labeling, once you have more than two single-sugar building
blocks, the compound is referred to as a carbohydrate and
not a sugar. On the food label, "Sugars" is the sum of the
single sugars plus the double sugars.

"Total Carbohydrates" on the food label includes the
single sugars, double sugars, sugar alcohols such as sor-
bitol and xylitol, complex carbohydrates, and fiber.

Further confusion comes about in the names of the sugars. Glucose, a single sugar, is the body's most important
carbohydrate and is referred to as blood sugar. On the food
label, however, glucose can also be called dextrose. Another single sugar, fructose—also known as fruit sugar
because it is the main sweetener found in (surprise!)
fruits—can also appear on labels as "levulose." (It is the
sweetest sugar—1.4 times sweeter than glucose.)

The most common double sugar, the granulated table
sugar you might use in your coffee, appears on labels as

"sucrose" or simply "sugar." It's made from one part glucose connected to one part fructose. Honey and invert sugar, which are also listed on the label, are made up of glucose and fructose, except they are not connected.

Other food sugars you might find include: lactose (milk sugar), which is made up of a glucose attached to another single sugar, galactose; maltose, a double sugar that is made from two glucoses attached to each other; and corn syrup, a sticky liquid that's primarily glucose plus some fructose. (There's also a high-fructose corn syrup, a sweetener in which fructose is the predominant single sugar.)

Sucrose = Glucose——Fructose
Maltose = Glucose——Glucose
Lactose = Glucose——Galactose
Glucose = Dextrose
Fructose = Levulose
Corn Syrup = glucose (mostly) and fructose
High-Fructose Corn Syrup = fructose (mostly)
plus glucose
Invert Sugar and Honey = glucose and fructose

The presence of different sugars in foods is not necessarily meant to mislead consumers. Rather, it usually reflects the different ways that food manufacturers use sugar other than as a sweetener. For example, sugar may be used to help inhibit the growth of microbes. Or it can serve as a food for yeast in dough-based products. Different sugars may be required for these roles, and each might have ended up with its own listing on the ingredient list. The new food labels have been able to cut through some of this confusion by listing the total quantity of carbohydrates and sugars per serving.

In addition, all types of sugar used to be listed together on the ingredient statement.

Glossary of Terms Used on Food Labels

Fat

Fat Free: Less than $1/2$ g (gram) of fat per serving (or per 50 g of food).

Low Fat: 3 g fat, or less, per serving (or per 50 g food).

Low in Saturated Fat: 1 g saturated fat, or less, per serving (no more than 15 percent of the Calories are saturated fat).

Percent Fat-Free: Contains the stated percent of non-fat ingredients. This term is allowed only in low-fat or fat-free foods.

Low Cholesterol: Less than 20 mg (milligrams) per serving (or per 50 g food).

Cholesterol-Free: Less than 2 mg cholesterol *and* no more than 2 mg saturated fat per serving.

Lean: Less than 10 g fat, less than 4 g saturated fat, and less than 95 mg cholesterol per 100 g ($3^1/2$ ounces). (Used on meat, fish, poultry, and game.)

Extra Lean: Less than 5 g fat, less than 2 g saturated fat, and less than 95 mg cholesterol per 100 g. (Used on meat, fish, poultry, and game.)

Milk Types

Reduced Fat, or Less-Fat Milk: formerly called low-fat or 2 percent milk; contains no more than 4.7 grams of total fat per cup.

Light Milk: Contains 4 grams of fat or less per cup.

Low-Fat Milk: formerly called 1 percent milk, contains no more than 2.6 grams of total fat per cup.

Fat-Free, Skim, Zero-Fat, No-Fat, or Non-Fat Milk: Formerly called skim milk, must contain less than 0.5 grams of fat per cup.

Calories

Reduced Calories: A product altered to contain 25 percent fewer Calories than the food it's being compared to. (Cannot be used if the other food already meets the requirement for a "low Calorie" claim.)

Calorie-Free: Fewer than 5 Calories per serving.

Low Calorie: 40 Calories or less per serving (and per 50 g food).

Light: Contains $1/3$ fewer Calories or $1/2$ the fat of the usual food. (If the usual food gets more than half its Calories from fat, the reduction must be $1/2$ the fat.)

Sodium

Sodium-Free: Less than 5 mg per serving.

Low Sodium: Less than 140 mg per serving (and per 50 g food).

Very Low Sodium: Less than 35 mg per serving (and per 50 g food).

Reduced Sodium: Contains no more than $1/4$ the sodium of the comparable food.

Light: Light can be used if the sodium content of a low-Calorie, low-fat food has been reduced by half.

Sugar

Sugar Free: Less than $1/2$ g per serving.

General Terms

Free: An amount small enough to have no likely effect on the body.

[Nutrient] Free: Food contains an insignificant amount of the nutrient.

Low: Low enough so that you can have it many times during the day without exceeding dietary guidelines.

Less or Reduced: Contains at least 25 percent less of the named nutrient than the comparable food.

More: Contains at least 10 percent more of the named nutrient than the comparable food.

High In: One serving must contain at least 20 percent of the daily requirement.

Source of: One serving must provide 10 to 19 percent of the daily requirement.

Healthy: Must be low in fat and low in saturated fat.

Fresh: Must be raw, and not frozen, processed, or preserved in any way (irradiation at low levels is allowed). Other uses, such as "fresh milk" or "freshly baked bread," are still permitted.

Fresh Frozen: Quickly frozen while still fresh (blanching before freezing is permitted).

Light: Can be used to describe properties such as taste, texture, and color, but the label must explain the intent, such as "light brown sugar."

More: One serving contains at least 10 percent or more of the Daily Value than the food it's being compared to.

Synonyms

Free: Without, no, zero.
Less: Fewer.
Light: Lite.
Low: Little, few, low source of.
Fresh Frozen: Freshly frozen, frozen fresh.

Implied Value

A product cannot claim to be made with an ingredient unless it has enough to be considered a good source of that ingredient. For example, "made with oat bran" can only appear on products that would be considered a good source of fiber.

Health Claims

The FDA is now permitting a number of health claims on the role of foods in reducing the risk of certain diseases. In order to make these claims, the food has to meet certain criteria. In addition, the language of the claim must always use words like *may* or *might* when discussing the connection between food and disease. The label must also state that other factors play a role in the disease.

There are nine different health claims that will be permitted on the label. The claims and requirements are as follows:

Calcium and Osteoporosis: One serving contains at least 200 mg calcium, which is 20 percent of the Daily Value. The calcium content must exceed the food's phosphorous content, and the calcium must be in a form that is readily absorbed by the body.

Fat and Cancer: The food must meet the requirements of a "low fat" food. If a meat, fish, or poultry product, it must meet the requirement for "extra lean."

Saturated Fat, and Cholesterol, and Coronary Heart Disease: The food must meet the requirements for "low saturated fat" and "low cholesterol." The fat content must fall under the "low fat" classification, and if a meat, fish, or poultry product, it must meet the requirement for "extra lean."

Fiber-containing Grains, Fruits, and Vegetables, and Cancer: Food must meet the requirements for "low fat" and be a "good source" of dietary fiber.

Fruit, Vegetable, and Grain Products That Contain Fiber, and Risk of Coronary Heart Disease: Food must meet the requirements for "low saturated fat," "low cholesterol," and "low fat," and must contain at least 0.6 g fiber per serving.

Sodium and Hypertension: Food must meet the requirement for "low sodium."

Fruits and Vegetables, and Cancer: Food must meet the requirement for "low fat," and must be a "good source" of at least one of the following: dietary fiber, vitamin A, or vitamin C.

Oats and Heart Disease: The food must contain at least .75 g soluble oat fiber (beta glucan) per serving. The products can have no more than 3 g fat per serving.

"Natural" Misconceptions

From scanning food advertisements, it looks as though foods are promoted for what they don't have more than for what they do: "no cholesterol," "no preservatives," "no additives." Considering our love affair with such negative attributes, it's ironic that a word as popular and positive-sounding as *natural* has no real meaning in food.

An official definition would have to come from the three governmental agencies that oversee the food industry, the most important one being the FDA. With the exception of meat and poultry products, which are regulated by the U.S. Department of Agriculture (USDA), the FDA is the agency charged with protecting our nation's food supply. Among other things, the FDA regulates the information appearing on food package labels. To date the FDA has defined all the descriptive terms that will appear on the new food label—all, that is, except *natural*."

The Federal Trade Commission (FTC) is the government organization that oversees food advertising in the printed and electronic media. In 1980, the FTC said that to be advertised as "natural," a food cannot contain any artificial or synthetic ingredients. In addition, a "natural" food can be no more than minimally processed. Although they've yet to iron down exactly what "minimal processing" means, the FTC, at least, has some semblance of a working definition.

The USDA also has a definition for "natural" that's in effect for all meat and poultry products. They say that a "natural" food can have no artificial flavors or colors, preservatives, or other synthetic ingredients.

Although the word *natural* remains undefined by the FDA, consumers apparently value the idea for their food. In a *Parade* magazine survey, 79 percent of those asked used "natural" as part of their definition of a healthy food. Given this level of interest, it's not surprising that manufacturers go out of their way to put "natural" on their labels. But without labeling regulations, manufacturers are free to take liberties with the term—and many do.

Fruit juices are good examples of "natural" deceptions. Food manufacturers take a fruit juice with a naturally high concentration of sugar, such as grape juice, and "artificially" strip it of all nutrient value but the sweetness. This stripped white grape juice, which is little more than sugar, is then used to sweeten foods sold as "all natural" 100 percent fruit juice. Naturally, this "all natural" shuffle adds to the price of the product.

Consumers assume they are getting all fruit juice, but often they're getting only a dose of sugar. Indeed, most commercial fruit juices sold as "natural" have grape juice listed near the top of the ingredient list—usually ahead of the juice whose name appears on the product label.

Regardless of how processed an ingredient might be, if it originates as a naturally occurring or living material, either mineral, plant, or animal, the ingredient can be called "natural." For example, some foods use corn sweetener, which is made by treating cornstarch with an enzyme that breaks down the corn's complex carbohydrate into individual sugar units. Because the sweetener began as corn, it's considered a "natural" sweetener.

Additionally, "all natural" doesn't mean additive-free. There are "natural" colors, flavors, and preservatives. But some of these ingredients would certainly challenge our "natural" sensibilities. For example, a widely used red coloring, carmine, comes from chemicals extracted from ground-up insect parts. But since the bugs are found in nature, carmine is called a natural color.

Simplesse is a fat substitute made from milk and egg proteins. This product is marketed as "all natural" because it started out as food. It doesn't seem to matter what form of processing is used, so long as the food starts out with a natural pedigree. There will even be room for biotechnology under this very large umbrella. As new food crops are developed through genetic engineering, if sold after only minimum processing, they also will be "natural" foods.

How unfortunate that *natural* is so misused and misunderstood. The consumer appears to like the idea of "natural" in the mistaken belief that this is a guarantee of wholesomeness. There are plenty of "natural" toxins that attest to this fact.

Until natural is properly defined, its presence on a label is nothing short of deceptive. As things stand now, there is no reason to believe that a processed food labeled "natural" is any more or less healthful than a similar product that does not use this word.

Shopping by the Labels

Before you decide on a product, examine the name, ingredient list, and nutrition panel. When deciding between products, study the labels side by side to see which offers more of what you seek.

Does one have fewer Calories from fat? Is one made with whole grains? Is sugar the number-one ingredient or is it farther down on the list? Is partially hydrogenated fat near the top of the ingredient list? Does one contain the vitamins and minerals you seek? You can, for example, identify foods with a higher percentage of Calories from fat by comparing the Calories from fat with the total Calories per serving.

And finally, before you toss your chosen brand into your cart, check the package for any defects such as water stains, leaks, or bulges that may indicate mishandling or tampering. You should also check for a freshness date to ensure you're getting a product that can be used before it expires.

The Label Can Only Do So Much

Although food labels can give you useful information, they are not the best tool for educating yourself about health and nutrition. The real strength of the label is to help you decide between items. You still need to understand the relationship between food and health. The basic knowledge will help you to form a nutrition agenda and shopping strategy. And in this context, the label can help you decide which products are best.

19. Food Additives

You may be shocked to learn that the average individual consumes about 140 pounds of food additives every year. That sounds like a lot, but of that amount about 114 pounds is sugar and about 15 pounds is salt. Other common food additives are corn syrup, citric acid, baking soda, vegetable colors, mustard, and pepper. With these you have accounted for about 98 percent of the food additives. The remaining 2 percent is there only in small amounts, but because of the labeling laws, these additives will be listed on the food label.

A food additive is any substance that is added to food. When a substance is added on purpose it is called an intentional food additive, or a direct food additive. An example of this would be the use of a preservative, a color, or a flavoring agent.

Substances can also get added to food unintentionally, however, say as a side effect of processing. These are called indirect or unintentional food additives. An example of this might be a chemical in the food's packaging that ends up in the food.

Whatever their source, food additives are strictly regulated. The testing of an additive can take several years, including a comprehensive battery of chemical and animal testing for a wide variety of potential effects. Finally, the Food and Drug Administration (FDA) decides on its safety and regulates its use in foods.

It wasn't always this way. For a long time there was little control over what was added. Unscrupulous food purveyors could get away with using questionable chemicals to make already-spoiled foods take on the appearance and taste of a more wholesome product. It wasn't until 1889 that a USDA chemist named Harvey Wiley began to examine the widespread use of additives. His work led to the Pure Food and Drug Act of 1906, the Food, Drug, and Cosmetic Act of 1938, and eventually to the Food Additives Amendment of 1958. These laws formed the protective framework that still remains in place.

Consider the fact that when we *process* foods by separating them into their constituent parts, and reassemble new foods with new sets of characteristics, we have to supply the taste, texture, consistency, and appearance. There also may be a need to maintain or improve the food's nutrient value, and to help maintain the product's freshness.

Speaking about freshness: What about food safety? Whenever there's a need to keep a food safe for an extended shelf life, some form of food preservation is required.

Nature has its own ways of protecting its foods, but how are we going to protect the foods we make? Usually, that involves processing the food in a way that will effectively stave off the particular type of breakdown that's most likely to occur. It is often done with the use of food preservatives, and in many cases we use the same types of additives that nature uses.

Unnatural Flavors—Artificial Fears

The tastes we associate with fresh, whole food come from distinct combinations of naturally occurring chemicals. The business of copying these flavors for use in processed foods involves a high-tech science complete with chemists and secret formulas—all designed to fool your palate into thinking you've gotten hold of the real thing.

Before a flavor can be copied, the chemists first need to identify the compounds that comprise the flavor in the genuine article. If the copy is to be an artificial flavor, all the chemists need to do is use synthetic versions of the natural flavor compounds and reconstruct the taste piece by piece. Where nature might use hundreds of chemicals in a particular flavor, the artificial copy may use only a small number—just enough to give the food a basic version of its intended taste.

If the copy is to be a "natural" flavor, the task is more complicated: The chemist has to combine different naturally occurring substances that, together, add up to the same flavor impression as the target taste.

Why can't food manufacturers make natural flavors with extracts from the actual food itself, such as using real strawberries to flavor strawberry Jello-O or strawberry ice cream? Although this direct approach might seem preferable, it's impractical on a large scale. As flavors go, the natural ones are typically weak in intensity. Many are unstable and break down during processing or storage. In addition, natural flavors may interact with other ingredients or even with the packaging material.

There's also a question of uniformity. While fresh foods grown by nature vary in flavor, processed foods must answer to a higher authority: the consumer. Biting into a fresh orange that tastes bitter won't stop you from eating oranges, but that same bitter taste in a processed food made with "natural orange flavor" might lead you to cross it off your shopping list for good. It's clear that the customer expects the taste of a processed food to be as uniform as its package. Even if scientists could control the vagaries of a pure flavor, the supply couldn't meet the demand.

> If manufacturers used real strawberries to make popular products such as strawberry Jell-O, the world supply of strawberries would be likely exhausted in a matter of days.

To meet the demand for natural flavors, chemists have to search for flavorful natural ingredients that work well in processed foods. They then catalog the different taste characteristics of each ingredient. When chemists are asked to copy a particular food flavor, they go to their catalog of natural ingredients and come up with a blend of flavors that mimics the genuine article.

These days, there's a strong desire by food marketers to have "natural" or "no artificial anything" on their label. It's questionable, though, what you, the consumer, gain from this.

Going back to our strawberry example, how much strawberry would you think is actually present in a food made with "natural strawberry flavor, with other natural flavors?" The answer may surprise you. Although there's probably a pinch of flavor from the actual fruit, it's likely that the bulk of the strawberry taste comes from other ingredients, such as bois de rose, a natural oil from the tropical rosewood tree.

Government regulations require at least some of the actual strawberry to call a food strawberry-flavored. It's unclear, though, exactly how much strawberry is needed, or whether anyone pays attention to the flavor formula so long as it tastes like strawberries. And by definition, the only requirement to call a flavor "natural" is that all the components come from natural sources. In the example, therefore, strawberries don't have to be a part of the flavor formula.

Ironically, one's sense of taste is not always the best way to identify a natural flavor. One product flavored with a higher percentage of real strawberries might actually taste inferior to another that had a better formula in its so-called "other natural flavors." Then, too, the natural flavors might not taste as good as the artificial flavors.

Check some labels next time you're at the store. Combinations of exotic ingredients—indicated on a package label by the innocent-looking words "natural flavors" or "with other natural flavors"—have become commonplace in processed foods. But with today's level of scientific expertise we can no longer assume that a product is more wholesome just because it uses natural flavors, or that it's inferior just because the flavoring is artificial.

Rather than relying on flavors from exotic substances, like oil from the tropical rosewood tree, artificial flavors can be made with synthetic versions of the exact flavor components found in the original fruit. This means that a natural flavor does not offer any taste or safety advantages over its synthetic counterpart and, likewise, because a food is synthetically flavored there is no reason to fear its safety.

> In Europe, they have a much more logical approach. They have a class of flavors known as "nature identical," which describes artificial flavors that only contain compounds that are chemically identical to those found in the real food. In the U.S., by contrast, there are no guidelines as to which flavor compounds can be used.

In the end, a good advertising campaign might persuade a consumer to try a product, but repeat business and ultimate success in the marketplace will depend on how it tastes. In today's marketplace, the only way to avoid the issue of flavoring additives is to stick with fresh foods.

Food Coloring: What Price Beauty?

Nature has a genuine attachment to color. One need only scan the variety of offerings in any produce department to fully appreciate this fact. Color is one of nature's most important forms of communication and we have come to rely on it as an integral part of our evaluation of food. The presence (or absence) of specific colors is seen as an indicator of wholesomeness or ripeness, and as a hint of flavors and textures. We do, in fact, eat first with our eyes.

It's not unusual for people to have a hard time with food when the colors are wrong. One study demonstrated that volunteers couldn't correctly identify strawberry flavoring when it was tinted green. And in a classic work on how colors can affect us, a group of people in the early 1970s was fed a meal of steak, peas, and french fries—but under lighting that concealed their appearance. At the conclusion of the meal, the room lights were raised to reveal blue steak, red peas, and green french fries. Despite assurances that the food was wholesome and that the coloring was only the result of added tinting, a number of volunteers became ill.

Colors have been added to foods for hundreds of years. It's gotten to the point where we expect color perfection and use this as a standard on which to judge a food's level of quality. It is this reliance, together with the marketing of perfect-looking food, that has made adding colors to processed foods necessary in the eyes of manufacturers.

Color manipulation, however, is not limited to processed foods. Oranges, for example, may sometimes be *colored* orange to hide the natural blotches of mottled green that are sometimes present when the fruit is ripe.

Once it was commonplace for food coloring to be used unscrupulously to hide the defects of spoiled merchandise. For example, small amounts of copper sulfate, now a known poison, were added to bring pickles to a brighter shade of green, and lead-containing dyes were used in the past to give candies their bright colors. It took the passage of the Federal Pure Food and Drug Act in 1906 to outlaw such practices.

Over the years many colors have come and gone. A notable case involved the 1976 ban of FD&C Red No. 2, also called red dye No. 2, a widely used food and cosmetic coloring. This color, as with many banned before it, was found to cause cancer in laboratory animals. This ban—which among other things yanked the red candies out of the M&M bag—focused public attention on the possible dangers from artificial colors, and likely was a key event in the industry shift toward the use of natural colors. (Incidentally, red M&Ms being sold today rely on a different dye, FD&C Red No. 40.)

When we add coloring to food, it's not a "natural" event. But to make this most artificial of processes seem more natural, food manufacturers are turning to colors from natural sources. Although the name might suggest differently, "natural colors" are rarely natural to the food in which they're used. Rather, they are color-rich chemicals that come from animal, vegetable, or mineral sources.

Natural red food color, for instance, can be extracted from beets or it can come from carmine, a crimson pigment from the shell of a Central American insect. Both are considered "natural" red colors, and are used in everything from fruit drinks to candy to strawberry ice cream.

Label terminology for natural colors can be quite confusing. If a natural color is not "natural" to the food in which it's added—as in the use of a beet powder used to tint strawberry yogurt—the food cannot claim to be naturally colored. But since the beet coloring is "natural" in itself, the yogurt could claim to have no artificial colors.

Whenever artificial colors are used they must be indicated on the label. Currently the only color that must be mentioned by name is FD&C Yellow No. 5, also called tartrazine. The FDA ordered this special mention after scientific research projected that as many as 100,000 people in the United States, including many aspirin-sensitive individuals, could have allergic reactions to the coloring.

The "FD&C" in the name of an artificial color refers to the Food, Drug, and Cosmetic Act, the 1938 legislation that gave federal authority to the regulation of the dyes used in foods, drugs, and cosmetics. The act also instituted a numbering system for the chemical substances used to color these goods.

Despite regulation, there continues to be a justifiable

controversy surrounding the use of food coloring. After all, their entire purpose is to change the colors of food to be more acceptable to the consumer. Manufacturers fear that if they were discontinued, few people would be interested in purchasing a white stick of margarine, a gray hot dog, a brownish-gray maraschino cherry, or a colorless cola—even if these are the real colors of these processed foods. Because the public persists in holding perfect coloring as an ideal, it's only "natural" that the consumer buys those foods that look best—no matter whether that look came from nature or science.

Preservatives to the Rescue: The Good, the Bad, and the Moldy

If your diet were made up entirely of farm-fresh foods, you'd have little need for food preservation beyond that supplied by a refrigerator. Most of us, however, aren't that fortunate. The alternative is to rely on food suppliers who are forced to cope with the reality that the nutrients in food are just as attractive to microorganisms as they are to us.

Whenever there's a need for shelf life, some form of food preservation is required. Usually, that means adding something to the food to stave off the particular type of breakdown that's most likely to occur.

Preservatives come in two basic groups: *antimicrobial preservatives,* which stop the growth of bacteria, molds, fungi, and yeast that can destroy food; and *antioxidant preservatives,* which prevent rancidity, off-flavors, and discoloration caused by the natural chemical reaction of oxidation.

As a group, preservatives get mixed reviews. Some are essentially harmless in the minute quantities used, particularly those based on natural substances.

In nature, vitamin E (tocopherol) is used to preserve plant

seed oils and vitamin C (ascorbic acid) is used to keep fruits and vegetables fresh. Both are natural antioxidants. Fruits such as cranberries, raisins, prunes, and citrus all contain naturally occurring acids that make effective antimicrobial agents. When used in foods, these compounds have last names like citrate, propionate, benzoate, sorbate, and lactate.

As an example, one such compound often found in breads, calcium propionate, retards the formation of mold. Food manufacturers can add calcium propionate directly, or use raisin juice, which contains propionic acid, the organic acid on which calcium propionate is based. In either case, these natural compounds and others like them are harmless at the levels used.

Some preservatives have an inconsistent safety record; noteworthy among these are *sulfites, synthetic antioxidants,* and *nitrites*. Although sulfites are effective antioxidants, the FDA estimates that as many as 100,000 people in the United States react to sulfite preservatives with symptoms like headache, hives, or shortness of breath. Recently, the FDA banned the use of sulfites on fresh fruits and vegetables (except potatoes). They are still used in beer and wine, but when present it must be indicated on the label.

Synthetic antioxidants commonly found in foods include BHA (butylated hydroxyanisole), BHT (butylated hydroxytoluene), TBHQ (tertiary butyl-hydroquinone), and propyl gallate. These preservatives are used because they are less expensive and more efficient than naturally occurring antioxidants like vitamin E. They have been cleared for safety through animal tests, but they are synthetics, and there's still a question of long-term safety and possible buildup in the body.

Nitrites are added to sausages, bacon, and other cured meats because they inhibit *Clostridium botulinum,* the bacteria responsible for botulism poisoning. In food or in the body, in the presence of protein nitrites can be converted into nitrosamines, compounds known to cause cancer in animals.

Nitrites and nitrates (which the body can convert to nitrites) are naturally present in several vegetables, including turnip greens, beets, celery, rhubarb, spinach, radishes, parsley, and lettuce. Nitrites are also found in beer and cheese. When you eat these foods and a protein food at the same meal, nitrosamines can be formed in your stomach, but the risk is minimal because of the presence of other nutrients, such as vitamins C and E, which help limit nitrosamine formation.

The risk from nitrites in cured meats, however, is different because all the ingredients needed to form nitrosamines are in the same package. The nitrites together with protein and a high cooking temperature make an ideal environment for nitrosamine formation. This means that the nitrosamine could already be formed when you eat your bacon or sausage.

In choosing between the possible dangers of botulism and nitrosamines, a government panel picked nitrite preservatives as the lesser of the two dangers. It was suggested, though, that consumption of nitrite-containing cured foods be limited. So if you're going to eat cured or smoked meats, the use of nitrite preservatives is a risk you must be prepared to accept. Although most smoked and cured meats contain sodium or potassium nitrite, you can find nitrite-free meat products either as locally made, short-shelf-life products, or in the freezer case where the low temperature effectively inhibits bacterial growth. (To be safe, however, these products should remain frozen until prepared.) Another option is to look for a product that also contains sodium ascorbate (a salt of vitamin C), sodium erythorbate, or vitamin E, as these antioxidants also inhibit nitrosamine formation.

Nitrates aside, it is important to realize that not all preservatives are cause for concern—especially ones based on naturally occurring substances. What's the value of preservative-free foods if half the product gets discarded, or worse, if you end up eating food that has already begun to spoil?

20. When the Fat Is Fake

Up and down the aisles of the supermarket we're seeing more and more shelf space devoted to new products with less fat in their formulas. Whether it's bakery, dairy, deli, or frozen foods, the battlefield for acceptance in this $3.1 billion-a-year field is your mouth. The campaign being waged is to fool your sense of taste into thinking you're eating the full-fat item.

How do most phony fats work? Do they represent good nutrition or do they only serve to confuse our need to make better food choices?

To replace the fats in foods, scientists had to identify how the fat contributed to taste. Usually, the role of fat has to do with "mouth-feel." This term refers to a slippery, slide-over-the-tongue sensation that coats the mouth and carries the food's flavor. To come up with practical fat substitutes, technologists had to find one or more ingredients that would give this sensation, carry similar flavors, and not add fat Calories to the product.

To replace fat, many companies turned to naturally occurring food materials. This made sense, as it's likely that any new synthetic substances would be closely scrutinized by regulatory agencies such as the FDA. No one wanted another ingredient that needed a warning label. The most versatile fat replacers, it turns out, have been found among the family of nondigestible dietary fibers.

Those fibers now being used as fat replacers or substitutes include vegetable gums such as agar agar, locust bean gum, tragacanth, xanthan gum, and pectin. Other fibrous fat substitutes include dextrins, gels, glucomannan, and carrageenan.

These harmless ingredients contribute no vitamins or minerals; they act as binding and thickening agents, adding texture and that slippery mouth-feel to such foods as yogurt, salad dressings, sauces, jellies, puddings, sherbets, and ice cream. Although they're built like a carbohydrate, they're not digestible so they don't contribute any Calories to the meal.

High-fiber fruits, it turns out, can serve as a fat substitute in some baked goods. Prunes and applesauce, for example, by virtue of their high content of "slippery" carbohydrates can directly replace some of the butter in recipes for cookies, muffins, and cakes. The fruit's water-holding fibers and carbohydrates help shore up the structure of dough and give the final product the needed mouth feel we've come to expect from the full-fat product.

Simplesse, Trailblazer, and Dairy-Lo are brand names for a type of protein-based fat substitute. These substances are able to perform their feat because they're made from proteins that are broken into minuscule particles that slide over one another and contribute fat's taste appeal without the Calories. We find these fat substitutes in refrigerated dairy products.

Rather than a fat substitute, a new ingredient called Caprenin is a formulated fat that provides fewer Calories. It is now being tried out in candy bars, including the new Milky Way II. Caprenin accomplishes its Calorie reduction by being made from fats that the body is not able to digest efficiently. As a result, a gram of Caprenin provides only 5 Calories, compared with the 9 Calories per gram we get from other fats. However, although you save a few Calories with Caprenin, it's still a fat, not a fat substitute. A modest gain, at best.

Another ersatz fat, called Z-Trim, was developed by the U.S. Department of Agriculture from a variety of low-cost agricultural by-products such as hulls of oats, soybeans, peas, and rice, or bran from corn and wheat. The hulls or bran are processed into microscopic fragments and purified, then dried and milled into an easy-flowing powder. When the fragments absorb water, they swell to provide a smooth mouth-feel. Since the product is made from natural dietary fibers, there is a minimal risk of adverse reactions.

If you're considering these products, it's important to keep in mind that although these products are safe, switching from full-fat fresh foods to fat-reduced processed foods is not the answer to good nutrition. Pseudo-fat processed foods do not measure up to nutrient-dense, naturally low-in-fat fresh fruits and vegetables. What's more, you cannot automatically lower your guard once you've switched to these lower-fat alternatives. Preliminary studies have shown that people who eat reduced-fat foods tend to compensate for lost Calories by having more to eat.

Olestra: A Slippery Fat-Free Fat

We have finally gotten to the point where we've toned down the polyester for the outside of our bodies, and now look what's happening. The Food and Drug Administration has approved a new polyester for the inside. The polyester here is sucrose polyester, which is the chemical name for the newly approved fat substitute Olestra.

Made from vegetable oil and sugar, Olestra looks like fat, cooks like fat, and offers the same rich taste and mouth-feel as real fat.

Naturally occurring fats in our foods come packaged in the form of triglycerides. All triglycerides share the same basic structure. They look like a squat version of the letter *E*. The "backbone" of the *E* is half of a glucose molecule called glycerol, and the three prongs are individual saturated or unsaturated fats.

Our bodies have digestive enzymes that are specifically designed to work on the triglycerides. These fat-digesting enzymes separate the fats from the backbone so they're small enough to pass through the absorptive surface of the intestines.

Where Olestra differs is that it is a synthetic molecule with a much larger sucrose backbone. It has six, seven, or eight fatty acids attached. This greater size confounds the body's fat-digesting enzymes, and the Olestra molecule passes through the digestive system intact and unabsorbed. That means zero grams of fat and no fat Calories.

As enticing as the idea of a fat-free fat may be, there's a worrisome side to Olestra that needs to be considered. Early problems with Olestra had to do with its unfettered trip through the digestive track. Aside from the potential for cramping and other digestive disturbances, the Olestra was found to bring about a condition known indelicately as anal leakage. That problem has been corrected to some degree, but intestinal distress is still a possibility. The FDA announced that Olestra would have to carry a warning label declaring this fact.

But what we don't see or feel, may represent the greatest concerns. The fundamental problem with Olestra is that it's made up of real fats. As it travels through our digestive system, other fat-based compounds that are present tend to mix with the Olestra. But the Olestra doesn't necessarily usher them *into* the bloodstream like other food fats; it can actually carry them out of the body.

At present, the established fat-soluble vitamins include vitamins A, D, E, and K. Olestra will be fortified with small amounts of these vitamins to, theoretically, take the place of any that might be pulled out of the system.

There are, however, many other fat-soluble assets in the foods we eat. The carotenoids are a family of compounds that continue to demonstrate their mettle. A study published in the *American Journal of Clinical Nutrition* found that a small serving of Olestra-prepared potato chips resulted in significantly fewer carotenoids being absorbed into the bloodstream.

Lycopene, a carotenoid compound found in tomatoes, has potent antioxidant qualities. And then there are the plant sterols, such as the soy isoflavone, genestein, which was recently associated with a decreased risk of cancer. More and more scientists are finding out what's in healthful foods that makes them so healthful. And, like the above examples, many of these compounds turn out to be fat-soluble.

If Olestra is eaten at the same time as any food containing a health-promoting fat-soluble compound, it has the potential of shuttling a significant proportion of that compound out of the body.

Are there any potential effects on fat-soluble medications? Many prescription drugs are made from fat-based substances. Steroids, hormone-replacements, birth control pills, and cholesterol-lowering medications, for example, are all fat-based compounds. Is it possible that these or other fat-soluble medications could be prevented from entering the bloodstream and carrying out their assigned tasks? If so, which ones are affected? And how soon before or after an Olestra-containing meal could such prescription drugs be safely taken?

The key, of course, will be the dose. The more Olestra-containing meals you have, the greater its potential effect. But answers to these questions should be available before the first Olestra-containing product appears on the supermarket shelf.

Snack foods are the first category that the FDA approved. But if snack chips are successful, can cooking oils and shortenings be far behind? And what about America's passion, the fast-food french fry? Olestra's finding its way into the french fryer would represent a financial bonanza for Proctor and Gamble.

> I don't favor the widespread use of Olestra. Health professionals are constantly counseling consumers to exert self-control over what they eat. It's these same consumers whose ever-expanding waistlines seem to shout that control over food selection is not their strong suit. A serving of snack chips is usually about one ounce, which translates to about fifteen chips. The lure of snack foods made with a "fat-free fat" could be too much for many to pass up.

I understand, however, the sentiment that Olestra should have a chance in the marketplace. Whatever your decision, keep in mind that an occasional serving of an Olestra-containing snack on an empty stomach will probably not do any lasting harm. Although upward of $200 million has been invested in developing Olestra, and great expense will be involved in marketing the products, the final arbiter of Olestra's success will be you, the consumer.

21. Food Safety

Most of us have experienced food poisoning. A mild case usually results in a queasy stomach, intestinal upset, and a general sick feeling. Often what people think to be a case of the twenty-four-hour flu is, in reality, the aftereffects of a tainted meal. But the symptoms can be much more severe. Indeed, bacterial food poisoning is likely to cause 7 million illnesses and more than 9,000 deaths this year. Rather than showing signs of going away, the problem is getting worse.

The villains are the bacteria, viruses, and protozoan creatures that contaminate food. It's not unusual for fresh food, especially animal products, to contain some of these microorganisms. The problem arises when a quantity of these bugs manages to hitch a ride into your body on a serving of food. The most common cause of food-borne illness is the mishandling of food after purchase. Whether at home or in a restaurant or other food-service facility, unsafe methods of storage and preparation increase the odds that problem-causing bugs will end up on your plate.

In most cases, symptoms of food poisoning include nausea, moderate to severe intestinal distress, fever, and a bloody stool. Depending on the organism involved, the symptoms can begin as early as a couple of hours after the meal (staphylococcal poisoning), or as late as a couple of days (campylobacter and botulism).

Botulism differs from other food poisonings in that the

toxin also affects the nervous system. In addition to intestinal distress, symptoms can include blurred vision, headaches, and difficulty speaking, swallowing, and breathing. This disease can be fatal, especially in the very young and the very old.

Some of the more common members of our rogues' gallery include:

Campylobacter jejuni: Unpasteurized milk, meats such as beef and pork, poultry, and fish are likely hosts. This bacteria is usually present in the animal's intestines, and contamination is usually the result of poor hygiene during slaughter and preparation for sale. Will be killed during cooking. **Usual onset after eating:** 2 to 5 days.

Clostridium botulinum: Usually a problem with improperly home and commercially canned or preserved foods. This bacteria is found everywhere and is usually present in the soil. The spores of these bugs produce the deadly toxin that causes botulism. Food-preservation techniques, such as canning, must include a heat treatment that lasts long enough to kill the botulism spores. **Usual onset after eating:** 4 to 36 hours.

Clostridium perfringens: This bacteria is present in the soil and it can be present in any raw food. It is also present in sewage and in the intestines of humans and animals. It is killed at a cooking temperature of 140° F. **Usual onset after eating:** 8 to 12 hours.

Entamoeba histolytica (Amebiasis): This protozoan creature lives in our intestinal tract and is present in human feces. Contamination occurs from consumption of polluted water or from foods grown on tainted soils. Destroyed with cooking. **Usual onset after eating:** 3 to 10 days.

Escherichia coli: Found in undercooked ground beef,

fecally contaminated water, some raw foods, and imported soft cheeses. This is believed to be the bacteria responsible for traveler's diarrhea. **E. coli 0157:H7** is a particularly virulent strain of *Escherichia coli* that was involved in a number of outbreaks associated with undercooked ground beef. **Usual onset after eating:** 4 to 9 days.

Giardia lamblia: This protozoa is associated with contaminated water and any foods made with giardia-tainted water. The organism can survive in moist environments and cool temperatures. Raw fruits and vegetables and ice cubes may be a problem in areas where giardia is present. Will be killed during cooking. **Usual onset after eating:** 24 hours to 25 days.

Hepatitis A: This bacteria is found in uncooked or raw shellfish. Hepatitis A is a communicable disease and infected individuals will have this virus present in their bodies. The virus can be transmitted through poor personal hygiene followed by hand-to-hand contact, or contact with a contaminated object. There are vaccinations available for hepatitis A. **Usual onset after eating:** 15 to 50 days.

Listeria monocytogenes: Found primarily in contaminated milk products, this stubborn bacteria also grows in soil, water, and plants, and it is found in raw meat, seafood, raw milk, and cheeses. This bacteria can survive and grow in cool, moist environments continuing to grow at refrigerator temperatures. It can also survive heat treatments such as pasteurization. Contamination is believed to come from animals, soil, and sewage. **Usual onset after eating:** 2 to 30 days.

Norwalk Virus: This virus does not grow or reproduce in foods. It is present in the feces of an infected individual, and then, in contaminated soils or water. If present in foods, it's there as a contaminant that's associated with poor personal hygiene. It is not easily killed through cooking. **Usual onset after eating:** 1 to 2 days.

Salmonella: Usually found in uncooked poultry products, eggs, unpasteurized milk, and raw meats such as beef and pork. Salmonella is often found in an animal's intestinal tract, and food can be contaminated during slaughter and preparation for sale. Salmonella is killed when exposed to a temperature of 165° F or higher for a few seconds, or a temperature of 130 ° F for a couple of hours. **Usual onset after eating:** 6 hours to 3 days.

Shigella: These bacteria, which cause dysentery, are spread by person-to-person contact, and through the consumption of contaminated food or water. Flies are also a potential carrier. The shigella bacteria can be found as a contaminant in deli foods, such as potato salad, milk, and other dairy products. The bacteria are killed by cooking. The spread is attributable to poor personal hygiene. **Usual onset after eating:** 12 hours to 4 days.

Staphylococcus aureus: Can be a problem with any food. Staph bacteria is normally present on our skin and inside our nose and throat. Food handlers can "infect" foods if, during an illness, they sneeze or cough on food or handle it with unwashed hands. **Usual onset after eating:** 30 minutes to 7 hours.

Vibrio vulnificus: This bacteria is normally present in coastal water and it does not usually cause problems in healthy individuals, though it does pose a risk for immune-compromised individuals. It is not a pollutant. It's often found in shellfish, but it's normally killed through cooking. **Usual onset after eating:** Up to 3 days.

What About Eggs?

The FDA estimates that salmonella bacteria is found in one in every 10,000 fresh eggs and recommends that you avoid eating raw eggs and any foods containing raw eggs. Eggs are considered safe from salmonella only when the yolk and white are cooked firm. Many food-service organizations and restaurants are now switching to pasteurized eggs to avoid this problem.

At first it was thought that eggs were contaminated with salmonella after being laid, possibly through a crack in the shell. It was later discovered, however, that the bacteria was present before the shell was even formed.

Fresh eggs are washed and sanitized before packing and need not be rewashed before use. They should be kept in their original container under refrigeration in a cold part of the refrigerator—not in the door. If uncooked, eggs can be safely kept for a few weeks. Hard-boiled eggs under refrigeration can be kept up to one week. In either case, though, quality declines somewhat with time. Obviously, the odds are against a single egg being contaminated—the American Egg Board places the likelihood of your finding an infected egg at about 0.005 percent (five one-thousandths of a percent)—but for individuals most vulnerable to the ravages of food poisoning, taking all precautions would be prudent.

Who's Most Vulnerable?

The severity of the poisoning is tied to the strength of the immune system, the body's defense against invading bacteria. In healthy individuals, most bouts of food poisoning pass quickly. But for those with an impaired immune system, such a malady can be life-threatening.

Those who tend to suffer the most are infants and toddlers, due to their undeveloped immune system, and the very old, in whom inadequate nutrition, poor blood circulation, or other health problems inhibit the proper functioning of the immune system. In both of these groups, a smaller amount of acid is produced in the stomach, which allows larger amounts of bacteria to survive digestion in the stomach.

Diabetics are also at higher risk for food-borne illness because their tendency toward higher blood-sugar levels makes their systems more conducive for the growth of bacteria.

Cancer patients, those with advanced liver disease, individuals who are HIV-positive, and transplant patients on immune-suppressant drugs all have a seriously disabled immune system that is unable to fight off food-borne bacteria. The group at greatest risk, however, is the one in which the very fabric of immunity is gone—those with full-blown AIDS. For them, even the slightest exposure can be disastrous.

As at-risk individuals are often under the care of others, it's vital that care givers have the proper training and education to prepare and serve foods safely.

Fighting Back

As ornery as these bugs can be, temperature remains their Achilles' heel. In general, bacteria tend to grow between 40 degrees and 160 degrees F. When chilled, bacterial growth tends to slow, and when heated to 160 degrees most are baked out of existence. The bacteria that causes botulism are stopped by acid, so high-acid foods such as tomatoes, citrus fruits, and pickled foods tend to be safe. These bacteria are also thwarted by nitrite preservatives, which is why sodium nitrite is added to all cured meat products.

Temperature Control

- Refrigerators should be set no higher than 40 degrees F, and freezers should be set at 0 degrees F.

- Frozen foods should be defrosted in the microwave or the refrigerator, not on the counter (and don't let juices drip on other foods).
- Foods should be marinated in the refrigerator.
- Fresh meats, poultry, or fish that will not be consumed for several days should be frozen immediately after purchase.
- Leftovers should be put in the refrigerator as soon as possible; to be safe, wait no more than two hours after the meal.

Cleanliness

Even if food is properly cooled or cooked, you still can get food poisoning from careless handling. This usually happens when cooked food comes in contact with hands, utensils, countertops, or other surfaces that have not been cleaned since contact with uncooked food. Here's how to reduce the risk:

- Wash your hands before handling food. Also wash hands, utensils, dishes, cutting boards, and countertops after contact with uncooked food.
- When grilling, use a clean plate to carry the cooked food, not the same one that held the raw meat.
- Sponges and towels can also harbor bacteria, so be careful when using these on surfaces that will be in contact with cooked food.
- Wear gloves when preparing food if you have cuts or sores on your hands.

Are Wooden Cutting Boards Safe?

The safety of a wood surface depends on the food being cut and how often and in what manner you clean the board. Wood is not the best material on which to prepare all food.

Although they're attractive, wood cutting boards can absorb liquids, and food particles can easily become imbedded. When this happens, the board is a potential breeding ground for bacteria. If wood is your surface of choice, however, there are steps you can take to help make it a safe cutting surface.

To control the absorption of fluids, the wood surface first must be seasoned with oil. Don't use vegetable oil, however; edible oils such as corn, soy, olive, and canola will turn rancid and affect food. Instead, use a nonedible oil such as mineral oil. There's also a product called block oil, made especially for seasoning wood butcher blocks.

After each use—especially with meats—the cutting board must be carefully cleaned. At the very least, this means using very hot water plus detergent. To ensure that the surface is germ-free, use a mild disinfectant, such as a bleach/water solution (the USDA recommends a solution of 1 teaspoon bleach per quart of water). Then rinse well.

If there is only one cutting surface available and it's wood, the potential for problems is greater. It's best to have a separate board for cutting meat; a good choice is hard plastic that can be easily cleaned or put in the dishwasher. Always keep in mind that food is only as clean as the dirtiest surface it touches. By separating meat from non-meat cutting surfaces, and adopting a good board-cleaning routine, you reduce the possibility of cross-contamination between foods.

A container serves as an effective barrier between the food and the air. A simple but important safety practice is to be sure to close the top or seal the bag immediately after use. Buying in smaller portions is another option; this prevents food waste, but the tradeoff is increased expense, more trips to the market, and more empty packages. Consider buying in bulk and then splitting larger packages into smaller portions which can sit tightly sealed in the refrigerator or freezer until needed.

A container must remain in good condition to be safely reused. The key points are cleanliness and a tight seal. Containers of fatty foods, such as spreadable cheeses, can be difficult to clean if the rim or any irregular surface can trap food particles. If you plan to reuse containers, be sure to scrub them well *by hand* between uses—dishwasher cleaning is unreliable because the temperature isn't always hot enough and the machine doesn't reliably remove dried-on debris. If you can't clean the container absolutely, don't reuse it. Over time, many containers crack or deteriorate to the point that they no longer provide a good seal and should be discarded.

Finally, always be cognizant of the fact that bacteria are everywhere—on our skin and clothes, in dirt, on countertops, and in all perishable food. The types of bacteria that cause food-borne illness aren't necessarily the ones that spoil food, so just because food looks good is no guarantee that it's safe. If this discussion of fighting food-borne illness has made you wary, that's good; food poisoning is a problem that, by and large, is under our control. It will only go away when we make it.

E. Coli and the Bad News Burgers

We seem to be hearing more and more about food poisoning outbreaks from tainted hamburger meat. In one brief outbreak in Washington state, Idaho, and Nevada, at least one child died and more than 400—most of them children—were taken ill.

The organism responsible for the fast-food hamburger outbreak, called *E. coli,* is a common family of bacteria. *E. coli* happens to be a normal inhabitant of the large intestines. We're not poisoned by our own *E. coli* because it's a more benign strain.

But even this relatively common strain can become a

pathogen. Most urinary tract infections are due to *E. coli*. Traveler's diarrhea is also believed to stem from *E. coli*. The type of *E. coli* responsible for the recent outbreak is different. Called *0157:H7* since its discovery in 1982, this uncommon bug is a dangerous and virulent strain of *E. coli*. It was believed to have gotten into the meat when cattle containing this rare strain were used to make ground beef.

The U.S. Department of Agriculture system of meat inspection is present at just about every step of the meatpacking process. The inspector, relying primarily on sight and smell, attempts to ensure that sick and diseased animals, as well as contaminated or unwholesome meat, are identified and excluded from the market. But the system, as presently configured, does not allow the inspectors to accomplish this goal.

For example, it's not unusual for an animal's bacterialaden intestinal contents to come in contact with the carcass during slaughter. If there is any fecal matter greater than 1/8 square inch (about the size of a pea) on the carcass, it's supposed to be cut off by the USDA inspector. This may sound effective, but the inspector has only about ten seconds to check the internal organs and inspect each carcass. So it's questionable how much contamination is actually identified, caught, and corrected. It's doubtful that any visual inspection could have caught the *E. coli* before processing.

A more reliable detection of bacteria, especially virulent strains such as *E. coli 0157:H7,* could be accomplished, but it would require more costly and time-consuming procedures. Clearly some reform is needed. One possible change would be to routinely screen cattle for *E. coli 0157:H7* before slaughter. But at present, the onus falls on the person preparing the food to provide a final barrier to contamination. For as ornery as these bugs can be, temperature remains their Achilles' heel. Even if this virulent strain is in the meat, if it is cooked properly (up to 155 degrees), the *E. coli* will be destroyed. At this temperature, the meat is steaming hot and gray in appearance, and the juices run clear. Aside from adequately cooking meat, there is currently no way to guarantee that all the bacteria will be killed.

Food Irradiation

I must confess that I am somewhat intimidated by the idea of destructive radiation, having been raised in the specter of nuclear war. Let's face it, the idea that we would allow our food to be exposed to radiation and that anything good would come from it is a challenge to one's instincts. The battle I have is that my logical/scientific mind tells me the irradiation of foods is OK, but there remains a voice inside that keeps whispering doubt. With that as pretext, let's answer some basic questions about what this technology can and cannot accomplish.

What Is Food Irradiation?

It is a process that briefly exposes food to a radiation source. The source can be a nuclear isotope or an electrical device called an electron accelerator. The amount used is enough to reduce the number of disease-causing microorganisms or insect pests that can destroy fruits, vegetables, or grains, and it can inhibit sprouting in root crops like potatoes.

How Does Irradiation Work?

The radiation makes subtle structural changes in the food as well as in the bacteria and pests that happen to be present. Compounds called radiolytic products and free-radicals are formed. There is evidence that when irradiation is carried out according to specifications, the level of these compounds is harmless. They were found to be no different from similar compounds that might occur in non-irradiated foods. When done correctly, irradiation leaves no toxic residue and does not affect flavor. The food does not become radioactive, just as we do not become radioactive when we have an X ray. There is some nutrient loss, though.

Is There a Need for Irradiation?

Certainly not for all foods. Recent events have foisted irradiation into the spotlight as a way to help prevent bacterial contamination of ground beef. It had been suggested as a way to control insects on fruits, vegetables, cereals, and nuts. Irradiation could indeed kill *E. coli 0157:H7,* but there would still be the risk of contamination after the food was irradiated. Consumers would still need to practice safe food handling.

Is an Irradiation Plant Safe for the Workers and the Environment? What Happens if Something Goes Wrong?

These are difficult questions to answer with any certainty. In this country, there is a track record for the sterilization of medical instruments by irradiation. Those in favor of irradiation claim it to be an excellent safety record, while irradiation opponents say the facilities represent a hazard to those in and around them. To make irradiation as safe as possible, the radiation dose must be correct and there must be enough checkpoints at irradiation plants to catch any equipment malfunction or human error before the food gets eaten. If a food is over-irradiated, the color, taste, texture, and odor will be seriously affected and the food can be caught and rejected. The argument against irradiation, simply put, is based on the belief "accidents will happen." Any potential for mishaps in an irradiation facility must be given serious consideration, not only for its effects on the food, but for the potential dangers to the workers and those that live around the plant. It will be up to government regulatory agencies to ensure that safety standards are maintained.

In Using Irradiation Are We Simply Trading One Risk for Another?

Yes. But if our only options entail risk, as in irradiation versus bacterial contamination, it is reasonable that this technology at least be considered. What appears somewhat questionable is whether these are our only alternatives. With *E. coli 0157:H7,* there may be other options. Some begin down on the farm with the identification and treatment of those animals that harbor these bacteria. Others might be with better screening at the meat processing plant to eliminate those samples containing the bad bacteria. At present meat inspectors have only seconds to visually inspect meat carcasses. Perhaps what we need is to give the meat inspectors the power and the tools to do their jobs more effectively. It will be an awesome task, given the fact the total consumption of ground beef in the U.S. is about 7 billion pounds per year.

Finally, is our way of processing and handling foods inherently dangerous? Does it have to be? Consumers often cast a blind eye toward food as long as it looks and tastes good. But now that meat inspection methods have been called into question and the almighty hamburger is at risk, alternative methods such as irradiation are being proposed. The bottom line is that safe food handling in the home will always be essential.

The Dark Side of Nature

Eating, like any other human activity, has its risks. But fast-food hamburgers notwithstanding, not all the riskiness in our food supply comes from bacterial contamination. In fact, some of the "danger" is there on purpose.

Nature equips many fruits and vegetables with the ability to produce a variety of chemical toxins that help ward off insects, bacteria, fungi, and animal predators. Although these natural toxins are meant to help the plants survive in their natural environment, if taken by humans in sufficient quantities, they can cause illness, cancer, or even death.

Have no fear. Eating fruits and vegetables is healthy, not hazardous. But a look at these natural toxins illustrates the point that it's the dose that makes the poison. Here are some examples:

- Potatoes can produce *solanine,* a bitter-tasting toxin that affects the nervous system. Solanine is produced when the potato is exposed to sunlight or allowed to sprout. It is most concentrated in the sprout, but it's also present in potatoes having a greenish tint to the skin. To avoid solanine, keep potatoes in a cool, dark place. Carefully cut away all sprouts and green portions before cooking, and discard any potatoes that taste bitter.
- *Cyanide,* a deadly poison, is naturally present inside the seeds of apples and the pits of apricots, peaches, cherries, and other fruits. There's no danger if you don't chew on the pits because the cyanide isn't released unless the pit is crushed. Lima beans and other legumes once contained cyanide compounds, but through selective breeding, commercial varieties were developed that no longer have this trait.
- Cabbage, mustard greens, cauliflower, and brussels sprouts contain *goitrogens,* compounds that prevent iodine from being used by the thyroid gland. Without iodine the thyroid cannot function normally and the condition called goiter results. Goitrogens are not a concern unless you have an iodine-deficient diet and the above foods are a major part of your daily menu.

With the advent of iodized salt and the wide distribution of ocean fish (another good source of dietary iodine), iodine deficiencies are no longer common.

- Shellfish such as oysters, clams, and mussels are poisonous at certain times of the year when they are invaded by a toxic algae during the event called the *red tide*. While they don't damage the shellfish, these microorganisms produce a paralyzing nerve toxin for which there's no known antidote.

- Honey, despite its wholesome image, can contain minute amounts of deadly botulism toxin. While the level is too low to threaten adults, children less than a year old should not be given this sweetener.

- Spinach and rhubarb contain *oxalates,* another toxic compound. One serving of rhubarb leaves (note that people usually serve the stalks, not the leaves) contains one-fifth the toxic dose of oxalates for humans. Spinach leaves and rhubarb stalks contain lesser amounts.

There's little in the way of government protection against such natural toxins. The only applicable law, the Delaney Clause, states that no substance known to cause cancer at any dose shall be *added* to foods. For example, safrole, a naturally occurring oil, was once part of the flavoring in root beer. After evidence was published that large amounts of safrole could cause live cancer in animals, this flavorful oil was banned as a food additive. This had no effect, however, on the small amount of safrole naturally occurring in nutmeg, star anise, mace, and cinnamon.

To put all these natural toxins in perspective, we need to understand that the body is well equipped to handle small quantities of many toxins rather than large amounts of a few. One potato, for example, poses little risk, but the combined solanine from over 100 pounds of potatoes might be enough to kill a horse.

Your best defense against natural toxins is to eat a variety of foods. With variety, not only do you limit your exposure, you provide the nutrients the body requires to maintain its defenses. And as the name suggests, natural toxins are part of nature; they are not to be feared so much as respected. If you labored to clear your diet of all fresh foods containing natural toxins, it's likely you'd be left with an empty plate.

Seafood Safety: Has that Fish on Your Plate Led a Clean Life?

Concerns continue to be voiced about the safety of eating fish. This is unfortunate because fish is high in protein, a good source of B vitamins, and relatively low in fat. Nutritional value, however, is not the problem. At issue are potential hazards from chemical and bacterial contamination.

The safety of fresh fish depends on two elements: whether the environment in which the fish was raised was clean and whether the fish was properly handled and refrigerated after the catch. These are valid concerns, but with a little information you can minimize your risk and enjoy your fish for the wholesome meal it provides.

In polluted water, contaminants enter the food chain with the lowest sea creatures, such as algae or plankton. These contaminants work their way up the food chain as the tainted organisms are eaten by small fish who then become a food source for a list of increasingly larger predators. The amount of contaminants in any fish depends on how long (if at all) they have lived in polluted waters, and on the pollutants (if any) in the organisms they've eaten.

Freshwater fish are natural inhabitants of bays, rivers, lakes, and ponds, many of which might have questionable water quality. Therefore, it is wise to ask where the fish was caught and to avoid fish of unknown origin. Deep-sea varieties generally don't pose a hazard if they've spent their life out at sea. Again, ask where the fish came from. In theory, commercial fishing is done at least twenty miles offshore—away from most sources of pollution. But those who engage in sport fishing should be knowledgeable about the waters in which they fish. The joys of landing a big one are easily outweighed by any potential health hazards from an unsafe meal.

Some fish have definitely led a clean life. These are fish raised on specialized farms in a controlled environment—usually a spring-fed pond—where they dine on a well-balanced, vegetable-based fish chow. This ensures uniform high quality. Most fish farms are routinely checked by state inspectors. Americans buy about ten million pounds of farm-raised fish every year. Types of fish most commonly raised on farms are trout, catfish, salmon, and crayfish.

The nutritional value of a farm-raised fish is similar to that of its free-range cousin. One exception, however, might be the oils in the fish. Ocean fish, such as salmon, dine on smaller fish, insects, and plants. These foods are sources of omega-3 fatty acids, the health-promoting oils for which salmon and other varieties of high-fat fish are known. As the salmon consumes its ocean diet, these beneficial oils become a part of its body composition. Fish raised on farms, however, dine on a controlled diet that contains little of the omega-3 fats; hence, the farm-raised fish will provide significantly less of these fats.

Handling Fish

If not handled and stored properly, a fish out of water becomes a breeding ground for unwanted bacteria. Ice can effectively inhibit bacterial growth, but it must be used properly. On the way to the store and while awaiting sale, whole fish must be kept on a bed of ice. If the fish are stacked on top of each other in a refrigerated display case, there should be enough layers of ice to ensure that all the fish are sufficiently cooled. Cut-up fish, such as fillets and steaks, should be kept in single layers on lined trays over ice to ensure that the flesh or/and juices don't come in direct contact with the ice.

Choosing the Best Fish

When buying fish, the burden falls upon you to find the right store. A good one gets its fish from reputable sources and has the trained employees and proper equipment to handle it safely. Here are some general guidelines:

- Fresh fish should always smell fresh.
- When buying whole fish, the eyes should be clear, not cloudy.
- There should be a sheen on the gills.
- If you press on the flesh with your finger, it should spring back.
- Fish should remain cold from the store to your home; ask for ice if it's a long trip.
- Discard questionable fish—especially if you detect any off odors or flavors.
- Handle fish like any uncooked meat, making sure you wash hands, utensils, and serving dishes to avoid cross-contamination between raw and cooked food.
- Before cooking, trim off fatty areas and dark meat under the skin; these are the areas where contaminants tend to accumulate.
- Cook fish thoroughly—until the flesh becomes opaque and flakes easily with a fork.
- Eat a variety of seafood—don't always eat the same type of fish.

Getting the Lead Out

Often heard in old gangster movies was the threat to
"fill 'ya full of lead." While it's doubtful the bad guys were
about to force chips of leaded-paint down the throat of some
hapless victim, the result would have been devastating.

Medical studies on the toxic effects of lead appeared as
far back as the 1920s. An extensive and wide-ranging li-
brary of scientific studies has accumulated since that time.
One paper connected the fall of the Roman empire with
chronic exposure to lead from their plumbing.

Lead is toxic whether it's formed into a bullet or used to
make the color of paint. But bullets and paint are not the
only sources of this metal. In fact, for most people, food
and drink are the main sources of lead. And what's more,
there are other nutrients in the diet that can help determine
how toxic that lead will be.

The dangers of lead continue to threaten growing bodies—
it is the number one environmental hazard for young children—
but it can play havoc with adults as well. When this tasteless,
odorless mineral enters the body, it enters the red blood cells
where it can interfere with the manufacture of hemoglobin,
the oxygen-carrying substance in the red blood cells. Lead
also can enter the brain, and it freely passes through the placenta to a developing fetus. The list of lead's health effects
includes kidney damage, harm to the nervous system, high
blood pressure, growth retardation, and a permanent im-
pairment of mental abilities. Lead is more toxic during periods of rapid growth: pregnancy, infancy, and childhood.

Lead is found everywhere, so it's not unusual for the
body to contain small amounts. In fact, our system can
eliminate this mineral, albeit slowly. Health problems begin when the intake of lead greatly exceeds the body's handling abilities.

Often overlooked in discussions about the dangers of

lead is the role played by the other nutrients in the diet. Two in particular—calcium and iron—can decrease the amount of dietary lead the body will absorb.

Calcium entered the picture when studies found that animals raised on a low-calcium diet absorbed more lead than those on a high-calcium regimen. The current belief is that lead is absorbed through the same path as calcium, so a higher dietary calcium reduces the opportunity for lead to enter the body.

About twenty years ago scientists discovered that a diet low in iron increases the amount of dietary lead the body will absorb. Someone suffering from iron-deficiency has a significantly higher risk of lead poisoning. The lead-iron connection has public health implications: Inner-city populations that have the highest incidence of iron-deficiency anemia are those that have the greatest exposure to lead.

It becomes apparent that any strategies to limit the danger posed by lead must include a healthy diet with recommended amounts of calcium (1,000 milligrams per day) and iron (18 milligrams per day).

Dietary sources for calcium include dairy products, green leafy vegetables, sardines and other small fish with edible bones, oysters, broccoli, dried figs and apricots, navy beans, tofu, almonds, brazil nuts, and blackstrap molasses.

Iron can be found in red meats, poultry, fish and eggs, nuts, seeds, legumes, dried fruits, some dark green leafy vegetables, and iron-fortified cereals, breads, and rice.

Sources of Lead

Beyond good nutrition, we have to control or eliminate the sources of lead in the diet. Here is a list of ways that lead can sneak into the foods you eat.

- Older or imported ceramic bowls, plates, or dishes may contain lead in their colors or glazes. Unless they've been cleared for lead content, avoid using them with foods.

- Leaded crystal is loaded with lead. Short-term, meal-time use may be acceptable, but don't store beverages in leaded crystal.

- Although domestic wine producers have switched to tin or plastic bottle caps, older vintages and some foreign wine bottles may still use lead foil. If there is any question, use a damp cloth to wipe off the top rim and neck of the wine bottle after you remove the cork, and wipe off the cork before you reinsert it into the bottle.

- Domestic cans are no longer made with lead, but many third-world countries continue to use the less-expensive lead solder for their canned foods. Until this policy changes, you should consider imported canned foods a potential source of dietary lead. Unfortunately, there is no reliable way to tell just by looking if the seams in a can are made from lead. If there's a foreign-canned food you treasure, test the seams with one of the lead test kits listed below.

- Although many companies have switched to a soy-based product, many inks used on food wrappers still contain lead. There's little danger if you keep the ink-side out of contact with foods, or rinse foods (a good practice under any circumstances) that have been in contact with the ink.

- Fish, especially shellfish, from contaminated waters can contain hazardous amounts of lead.

- If the water pipes in your house are made from lead or contain lead solder, your tap water can become a major source of dietary lead. Hot water is more a problem than cold, and soft water leeches more lead than hard, high-alkaline water. Use only cold water for drinking or food preparation. If you need water after the taps have been idle for several hours, run the water for a couple of minutes, or until you feel the temperature turn cold, suggesting that fresh, outside water is now in your pipes. (You can collect the water you run off for non-food uses.) Another option is to use any of a number of water filters designed to trap lead. There are a number of inexpensive filter systems that rely on a water pitcher with a filter insert.

- Food from soils containing lead do not represent a serious risk. Lead does not easily dissolve, so it is not readily taken up by plants. Such food, however, must be thoroughly washed before eating to remove any possible leaded soil or dust on the skin.
- There are several ethnic home remedies that contain very dangerous levels of lead. The list of unsafe remedies includes: Azarcon or Greta (Hispanic); Pay-loo-al (Hmong); Kohl (Arab); and Ghasard, Bala Golo, and Kandu (Asian Indian). Some of these powders contain up to 70 percent lead. Anyone exposed to these remedies should seek medical attention immediately.

The main storage areas for lead are the bones and teeth. In one series of studies, scientists collected and analyzed the lead content of baby teeth to measure the extent of a child's lead exposure. Scientists discovered that cows allowed to graze on lead-contaminated pasture land will have elevated levels of lead in their bones. This is one reason that bone meal, a once-popular calcium supplement, is now considered unsafe unless cleared for lead content.

You can purchase lead test kits for use in the home from Hybrivet Systems (1-800-262-5323), or Frandon Enterprises (1-800-359-9000). Find out which is suited to the type of material you intend to test.

To test for lead in water, contact the National Testing Laboratory (1-800-458-3330) or the U.S. Environmental Protection Service water safety hotline (1-800-426-4791) for a list of certified laboratories in your area.

22. Biotechnology Heads to the Market

Most people have heard of biotechnology, but have only a vague idea of what it is. To some folks, biotechnology is a new way to improve the food supply, our health, and the environment; to others, the very idea evokes fearful images of unknown dangers from bizarre creations. Whatever your views, one thing is certain: This important new technology is coming, and it's vital that you understand what's at stake.

Our bodies are made up of millions of cells that all look remarkably similar when they're first created. Inside each cell is a set of instructions, or genes, that commands it to become the type of cell it's supposed to be. Biotechnology makes use of genetic engineering, or gene splicing, a technique that makes subtle changes in these instructions. The process can add to or change functions in a cell with a speed not previously possible. The changes, once made, remain a part of the cell that gets passed on to future generations.

You can begin to appreciate biotechnology's tremendous potential by looking at its use in agriculture. In the past, improving a food crop via plant breeding was a hit-or-miss process that took years to achieve any measurable success. Biotechnology removes much of the guesswork by identifying the specific genetic code associated with a desired trait. This code is then added to the genetic instructions of a target plant.

For example, the gene for good taste in plant A would be added to the genes of plant B, a variety with poor taste but a longer shelf life. From that point on, future generations of plant B would have a better taste *and* a longer shelf life.

Biotechnology has the potential to create crops that are less dependent on chemical fertilizers and pesticides, and are tastier, more nutritious, and have a longer shelf life. Many grains, for example, would be excellent sources of protein if not for the fact that they were missing an essential amino acid. Through biotechnology, the ability to add missing amino acids to grain, could turn inexpensive, easy-to-grow foods into sources of complete proteins. Plants might also be modified to grow in soil and water conditions where they previously could not survive.

Such a development would have little impact in the United States, where we already eat too much protein. It could, however, be a lifesaving change to developing countries where single grains are often the main food eaten.

Biotechnology can also produce crops that remain fresher longer. Unless you shop at farmers' markets, or a store that buys directly from nearby growers, the produce you eat has been picked unripe in order to get it to market before it spoils. With few exceptions, when produce is picked before ripening it will never develop a home-grown flavor. Varieties made through biotechnology would ripen on the vine and then last long enough to get to the store.

Biotechnology can also give us more options in food processing. For example, lactose intolerance, the inability to digest the carbohydrate in milk, can cause digestive problems in about 70 percent of the world's adults. Through genetic engineering, a bacteria could be developed that would digest the lactose in a fluid milk.

With such power and potential, the question of safety arises. Now that science has begun work on reprogramming the way things grow, is it just a matter of time before a mistake is made that opens a Pandora's box of new diseases, bugs, or even super weeds? Although unlikely, the possibility does exist.

There is government supervision of biotechnology through the FDA, EPA, and USDA, but there is little practical control over experiments conducted in individual laboratories. As experiments continue, a host of questions need to constantly be asked: Is this research necessary? Will this development feed more people? Will it provide a higher quality of life for a greater number of people? But who is going to ask these questions? And who will determine the answers? It is because of these unknowns that at this point biotechnology should be regarded only with cautious optimism.

Unfortunately, as great a potential as biotechnology may have, the forces that may decide its future will be those who control the purse strings of research. Government coffers are running dry and those of private companies are usually salted with economic self-interest, a fact that may not coincide with the good of humanity.

As an example, biotechnology can be used to make food crops that are resistant to a particular pesticide or herbicide. By growing these varieties, more chemicals could be applied to kill more pests without also killing the crop. Rather than a step toward less dependence on synthetic chemicals, such "advances" provide further rationale for their use. This development would not bode well for the environment. If biotechnology is used only for its profit-making potential, there's a real danger that the long-term health of the land and those who work it will become of secondary importance.

Few could argue with the use of this science to create varieties of plants with higher nutritional quality, a higher resistance to disease, or greater tolerance to variations in soil and temperature conditions. Such developments could change unfertile regions into productive farmland. This would be invaluable for those parts of the world constantly besieged by drought and famine.

However, will biotechnology chart a course toward the betterment of humanity, or will the science become just another industrial tool to use and abuse in the interest of profit? It's in your best interest to follow this field and make your opinions known with your voice and pocketbook.

PART IV

Bringing Home the Power of Food

23. Understanding What Science Has to Say

Although we all have a vested interest in their contents, most of you have neither the time nor the inclination to read scientific journals. If you did, you'd find yourself immersed in abstract abbreviations, methodological meanderings, and statistical slang. For those uninitiated in the prose of science, it is not what you'd call page-turner material—even though the contents often have a direct impact on your life.

But why even bother with the scientific journals when you can get your information in a much more user-friendly format? The printed and electronic media stand poised to report science's headier revelations alongside the daily weather and traffic report.

The reporting of science, it turns out, is more complex than can be contained in a paragraph or a sound bite. Despite its assumed objectivity, the conduct, reporting, and interpretation of science is far from dispassionate. There are personalities, varying abilities, and ego-bred self-interest at every step from the laboratory to the front page, all potentially conspiring to color our perceptions of what's going on and what, exactly, you need to do about it.

Here are some tools to help you decipher science. First, I'm going to give you a critical appraisal of how the media are doing as communicators of science and then give you some tips on how to be a better media science consumer. I have included a primer on the lexicon of science, those key words that reveal the relative significance of any particular study. And finally, I'll tell you how science goes to press, the role of funding, and what a study looks like, in case you want to read a journal article.

How Science Fares in the Media

On the surface, the idea of learning about science through the media makes sense. We've all got a stake in what goes on in the laboratories throughout our nation—aside from the fact that a large share of that research is funded with our tax dollars—and television, radio, and newspapers go into just about every home.

While relying on the media to deliver science's latest offerings sounds great, too often the messages are flawed. The problem stems, in part, from the fact that in the areas of nutrition and health, there is a yawning gap between scientific research and public understanding. That means that before the public can read or hear about science, it must first be put into a format that attracts attention and is easily understood. Most of us do not have technical educations, so regardless of the complexity of the research, the science reporters have to keep it simple. But while necessary, this can be a source of problems.

For example, recently there was a headline-grabbing story that reported how beta-carotene raised the risk of lung cancer. It was a bit much to swallow, since beta-carotene, the carrot-colored compound found in many vegetables, has been associated with a *decreased,* not an increased, risk of many cancers. Nonetheless, the story hit the headlines, based on a study published in the 1996 *New England Journal of Medicine*.

The study involved the use of beta-carotene supplements for a six-year period. But the stories gave short shrift to the fact that those in the study had been smokers for an average of thirty-six years before the study began. Lung cancer, it turns out, can take decades to develop, but once diagnosed it has a low survival rate. Beta-carotene, whether in supplements or in food, has never shown an ability to remove a cancer once it's already set up shop in the body—especially one as virulent as lung cancer.

And then there's the question of diet. The study was based in Finland, where the northern location makes for a very short growing season. The Finnish diet is not what you'd call a paragon of healthfulness, being marked by an excess of fatty foods and alcohol and a shortage of fresh fruits and vegetables.

Clearly, the journalists didn't ask the right questions and the misleading headline compounded the misunderstanding. It wouldn't have been fodder for front-page headlines, but the story should have read: "Men who are heavy smokers, who have smoked for many decades, cannot protect themselves from lung cancer merely by taking beta-carotene capsules for six years."

Competition Can Breed Confusion

Most people are unaware that there's an undercurrent of competition for the attention of the press. Front-page coverage can bring prestige, program funding, or, in the case of organizations, new members. Universities and scientific groups have therefore intensified their media outreach. Many journals offer advance copies to the press so that stories will be ready by the publication date. In 1990, the *Journal of the American Medical Association* (JAMA) actually advanced its weekly release date to the day before that of the *New England Journal of Medicine* (NEJM). At the time, JAMA editor Dr. George D. Lundberg stated in a *Los Angeles Times* interview that he wanted JAMA to be the first journal to publish new findings.

Competition for press attention within the science field

can play havoc with science coverage. The result is that media assignment editors are inundated with potential stories—many claiming broad importance for stories of limited scientific worth—but few editors and reporters have the science background to know which are really newsworthy. Articles in prestigious periodicals like JAMA and NEJM have instant credibility, but publicists for other publications have to pitch harder.

What makes this deluge of press releases worse is the scarcity of trained science reporters. Out of the almost four hundred schools of journalism in this country, only about twenty offer curricula in science journalism. Reporters with a limited science background can't look critically at a story on the basis of scientific merit. This knowledge gap can result in simplistic or sensationalist explanations of complex research concepts.

The selective reporting that results can sway readers dramatically—often in inappropriate ways. For example, after taking a fast track to food fame, oat bran experienced a precipitous drop in popularity following a media report casting aspersions on its reputation. The report in question came from a journal study that said oat bran was no better than low-fiber wheat flour. Left out, however, was the fact that the study's subjects were young and middle-aged women with normal cholesterol levels. By contrast, most of the studies that established oat bran's cholesterol-lowering ability were performed on older men with elevated cholesterol levels.

The study concluded that oat bran has little effect on young women with normal cholesterol." That message communicated to the public became "Oat bran has little effect. . . ."

Not Letting the Facts Get in the Way of a Good Story

One factor that works against accuracy is the journalist's desire to engage the audience. Whether writing for the printed or the electronic media, writers are never paid to bore their readers. How useful is information that isn't read? Writers need to aim, however, for a compromise between a boring article and a piece that thrills, scares, or outrages the public beyond objective justification.

Science can make good press whether the source is a research journal or a food safety watchdog group. Many times, though, a reporter will not even have read the study, but base their story on press releases that may or may not present a balanced view. Not all science fares well when force-distilled down to a headline and a few paragraphs.

As with the beta-carotene and oat bran stories, critical details are often lost and research conclusions taken out of context. Overworked reporters looking to flesh out the story consult only the most quotable or most accessible scientists and public understanding of science comes down to who or what sounds more convincing.

Evaluating Science Coverage

For major media, having staff with science savvy is critical. Reporters and editors with limited science background should constantly strive to improve their sources. News editors should keep science reporters in the loop. They can provide perspective on a story's scientific worth or potential local angles. A science advisory board or an unbiased consultant with science expertise can help sort through potential stories.

How can you better evaluate the science stories you read? Here are some steps to take and questions to ask yourself whenever you see a story:

• Read the entire article. Key qualifying facts are often placed near the end of the story. If possible, find versions by different authors in other publications. Check for similarities and differences.

- If the story represents preliminary evidence, is this fact emphasized or buried?
- Are both sides of an issue presented?
- Journals are not sold on the newsstand but are sent out via mail, so most scientists won't yet have seen a study at the time it's covered by the press. It's important, therefore, that the quoted sources have particular expertise in the topic area. Do you consider them to be unbiased?
- In a population or epidemiological study, which looks at risk factors and associations between behaviors and diseases, you need to consider whether the population studied is relevant to your location and lifestyle. (Remember the Finish smokers.)
- If the story is based on a survey, does the story make unwarranted comparisons or assumptions to formulate their conclusions?
- Who funded the study? The fact that a company has paid for a study that favors them doesn't automatically compromise the study's worth. Companies aren't going to spend their money on research that makes them look bad. There's additional assurance if the results appear in a peer-reviewed journal, for then the methods and conclusions will have been critically examined by other experts in the field. It always pays, though, to look at what else the scientist involved has done. Caution may be indicated if all his or her work follows the same basic theme.
- Pay attention to who's writing the story. By routinely making note of bylines you can begin to determine if the author is a science writer or a general reporter on a science assignment.

Finally, it's never a good idea to make wholesale changes on the basis of one study. If the finding is particularly relevant to your life, try to find out if this is the first study with this type of information, or merely the first one that makes it to the front pages.

The coverage of science is a difficult beat—one that by definition is subject to endless inquiry, debate, and revision. Once you begin to look critically, you will soon learn which publications and writers tend to rely on sensationalism, and which ones you can trust. In addition, you will develop the ability to pull key facts out of any story by separating the objective from the subjective.

How a Study Is Born

A researcher's status at his or her university and in the scientific community rests to a great extent on getting published. The more prestigious the journal in which the work is published, the more prestige the researcher gets.

Funding plays an integral role in determining how science progresses. Scientists need money to keep their research programs operating, and there's tremendous competition for a diminishing supply of research funds. To receive a research grant, a scientist submits an application that seeks to show the importance of the study being proposed. This usually means submitting existing scientific theory and publications on the topic, along with a detailed justification for the value of the proposed research. A decision is then made by a panel of scientists familiar with the field.

Because of this process, research proposals that follow along respected lines of inquiry are far more likely to receive funding than those that leap into new, unconventional areas. For better or worse, science tends to progress in small, studied steps that acknowledge and build on present understanding. This fact contributes to the generally conservative nature of scientific research.

After receiving funding and completing the research, the researcher writes a manuscript and submits it for publication. There is no rule that says they have to write up the study, but failure to do so may impact their ability to attract future funding. Once submitted, the journal sends the manuscript out for peer review, a process in which several scientists with expertise in the area assess its soundness and importance. The manuscript is not accepted for publication until the reviewers are satisfied that the methods and conclusions are valid and worthwhile.

The peer review committee may accept the manuscript, ask the researcher to do more work on the manuscript or collect more data, or reject the manuscript. Prestigious journals receive the most submissions and tend to the most particular about the research they accept. Factors that influence their decisions include not only the quality of the research, but also the author's reputation, the institution, and the popularity of the findings. While science is meant to be a dispassionate look at the facts, peer review boards are composed of people who bring their own biases to the process.

If the manuscript is rejected, the researcher may submit the manuscript to another journal. Researchers usually begin with the most prestigious journals and then move on to ones that are less critical. Unless the research or manuscript is seriously flawed, the researcher is likely to find a journal that will accept it. Be wary, however, of research findings from newsletters or popular magazines; they may be based on opinions or anecdotal evidence and not the result of a rigorous research study. Even major findings that are announced at scientific meetings may later be modified as the research goes through the peer review process prior to publication in a scientific journal.

A Guide to Study Terminology

Anecdotal Evidence, Personal Testimonial: Research based on casual observation, not rigorous scientific investigation. It may be valid, but it isn't proven. Anecdotal evidence is valuable because it can suggest possibilities that can be investigated in a more rigorous manner. For example: After suffering with a cold for a few days, you begin taking a new tonic. The cold disappears the next day and you're convinced that the tonic was the key. In this circumstance, however, it's impossible to say whether it was the tonic or if the cold had simply run its course. (Most colds do, you know.) Therefore, any claims that the tonic was a cold remedy would be based on anecdotal evidence.

Blind, Single Blind: Controlled research in which the subjects don't know whether they are receiving the treatment or a placebo.

Clinical Study: A study that uses people as the subjects.

Controlled Experiments: A form of research that can uncover cause and effect. The researchers use groups that are comparable in all aspects except for the treatment being tested. The "control group" gets no treatment. Therefore, any differences that occur between the groups can be attributed to the treatment.

Control Group: The group of subjects in a study not receiving a treatment.

Correlation: A relationship between two factors. If one increases when the other increases, these factors are said to be positively correlated, and if one decreases when the other increases they are negatively correlated. For example, if the incidence of heart disease goes up with an increase in blood cholesterol levels, it could be said that heart disease is positively correlated with one's blood cholesterol. This doesn't mean that cholesterol *causes* heart disease. The presence of a correlation doesn't mean that one factor causes the other, it just describes the relationship the factors have with each other.

Crossover Design: An approach in which the subjects in an experiment are given each of the treatments being studied, at different periods. For example, during a ten-week study of the acceptance of a diet pill, researchers gave half the subjects the pill and the other half a placebo. At Week 6, the treatments are switched. This design often gives more reliable data because the effects of the treatment and placebo are recorded for every subject.

Double Blind: Neither the subjects nor the researchers are aware of which treatment is being used. This approach provides the greatest precision because it removes any possibility of experimental bias.

Embargo Period: The period between when a scientific journal accepts a paper for publication and the paper's actual publication date. Traditionally this is a blackout period during which the authors cannot discuss their research findings with the press. If an author violates the embargo by "leaking" the finding to the press, the journal could penalize the author by refusing to publish the article or future papers from that author. Embargo periods can be anywhere from one to eighteen months depending on the backlog at a particular journal. Many journals send out press releases or prepublication copies of the journal when the publication date approaches. This allows the press time to conduct interviews and prepare stories.

Epidemiological (Population) Study: Observation of a defined group to investigate the relationship between health or illness and specific variables such as diet, activity level, or genetic history. The variables selected are usually those that are suspected of playing some role in the cause of the disease, but sometimes researchers collect information on a wide variety of variables in the hopes of discovering a relationship between previously unconnected occurrences. Epidemiological research can help suggest what's going on, but it can't explain a cause-and-effect relationship. Sometimes events that seem to be linked truly are; other times, the connections are coincidental. Only after numerous studies yield similar findings can you begin to come to any conclusions. An example of this is the epidemiological study discussed in chapter 21 that found that inner-city children suffering from anemia were at higher risk for lead poisoning. There was a connection, but did the anemia cause the lead poisoning or was it the other way around? Further research discovered that low blood iron causes the body to absorb more lead. Another example: While collecting data on airplane fatalities, it was found that physicians who eat more meat and consume more alcohol have one-third the risk of dying in a plane crash. Although one would have little problem finding volunteers, there wasn't much scientific interest in doing any follow-up studies.

Experimental Bias: Behavior by researchers that can influence the outcome. This does not necessarily involve dishonesty; it may be caused by the researchers' unconscious desire for or expectation of certain results.

Experimental Data: Information collected during a study.

Experimental Group: The group of subjects receiving the active treatment.

Manuscript: A scientific article submitted for publication in one of a number of formats. It can be a research study that presents new data, a review article that relates the findings of previous research, or an editorial or commentary that expresses an opinion about a particular topic.

Non-Refereed, or Non-Peer Reviewed Publication:

A publication that does not require its articles to undergo a peer review before accepting them for publication. Such publications may have scientific-sounding names, but the findings or claims that originate in such publications may be suspect. The articles may contain factual information, but the data have limited value when used as scientific proof. Popular magazines and newsletters are, as a rule, non-peer-reviewed.

Peer Review: A process in which a research article undergoes critical review by scientists having expertise in the area. The research article is not accepted for publication until the reviewers are satisfied that the methods and conclusions are valid and worthwhile. To satisfy the reviewers, scientists are often called upon to edit their submission or perform more tests. The journal editor usually has final authority whenever disagreements arise between author and reviewer.

Placebo-controlled Experiments: An experiment in which the control group receives a placebo. A placebo is a treatment that appears identical to the real treatment, but contains none of the active ingredients being studied. Using a placebo helps eliminate results that may be due to the subject's expectation that something is supposed to happen.

Prospective Study: A type of epidemiological study that looks at events and behavior in a correlation, then follows the group over the years to see what they do and what differences develop. Such studies are more likely than retrospective studies to generate scientifically valid results.

Randomized Design: Selected volunteers have an equal chance of ending up in either the treatment group or the control.

Refereed, or Peer-Reviewed Journal: A publication in which the research articles are required to undergo peer review as a condition of acceptance. Examples would include *New England Journal of Medicine, Journal of the American Medical Association, American Journal of Clinical Nutrition, Journal of the National Cancer Institute, Science, Lancet,* and *Journal of the American College of Nutrition.*

Research: A scholarly or scientific investigation. The term doesn't mean much in and of itself; it depends on the type of research and how well it was conducted. For example, someone trying to convince you to buy a certain product might say that it's "research-based." You don't really know if the "research" came from keeping notes, from reading a book full of unsupported ideas, or from articles that were published in a scientific journal.

Retrospective Study: A type of epidemiological study that looks at events and behavior that have already taken place. This type of study suggests connections but can't prove them or their relationship.

Risk Factor: Anything that has a statistical relationship with the incidence (but isn't necessarily the cause) of a particular disease. For example, having a high blood cholesterol level is a risk factor for heart disease, but not everyone with elevated cholesterol ends up with heart disease. In addition, risk factors vary in their importance. For example, it would be frightening to learn that your favorite food may double your risk of cancer. But if you found out that the odds of developing the disease increased from one in a billion to two in a billion, you probably wouldn't change your eating habits.

Significant Difference: An association or correlation that cannot be mathematically explained away as occurring by chance.

Survey: A collection of information from a small, representative group that permits conclusions about a larger population. Surveys may or may not have been conducted or critically reviewed by scientists trained in this form of study. Surveys offer a rapid and convenient way of gathering information, but what they offer in speed, they lack in precision. Size of sample, data collection methods, wording of questions, and other factors can greatly influence results.

Getting Through the Journal Jungle

If you brave reading a scientific study, you'll get a much more complete idea of the findings and their limitations. The following descriptions of the standard sections of a research article (roughly in order of appearance) should help you focus on the areas that contain the information you'll need. Check to see if the journal has any editorials on your topic, as these can offer additional perspectives on the findings.

Abstract: A quick take on the study, explaining what was done and what was found. It glosses over the fine points and says nothing about the study's flaws, limitations, or implications.

Key Words: Topics that help categorize the study. Useful when searching through a database.

Introduction: Explains why the study was done. Usually includes a brief historical review of what is known in the area, a statement of where the gaps in our understanding lie, and an explanation of how this research will contribute needed information.

Methods: An explanation of how the experiment was designed, the number and type of subjects covered, how they were selected, and how the study data were analyzed.

Results: An objective analysis of the collected information including tables and figures that graphically display the data.

Conclusion, Discussion: The conclusions justified by the results, explained in light of current knowledge and qualified by any limitations of the study. Researchers usually point out that theirs is not the final word on the subject and call for more research on the topic. If the journal allows editorializing, this is where it would appear.

Funding: In some journals, there are a few sentences telling where the money came from to conduct the study.

References: A list of all the scientific papers that were cited in the article. Depending on the journal format, they will either be listed alphabetically or in their order of appearance in the paper.

24. Avoiding Health Fraud

It's all a game of "Who do you trust?" Consider this:

The cover of a popular health magazine boasts that its contents can help you shed chronic fatigue, clear your sinuses, fall asleep faster, whip depression, hush your heartburn, escape computer ills, control diabetes, chop your cholesterol, and buff up your memory. That's quite an impressive line-up for the $1.95 cover price. Such bargains are far from unusual. They're all a part of the constant flow of ideas, theories, and claims that compete for our attention and acceptance.

In the check-out line at the food store, the tabloids call out with dramatic headlines of "amazing" or "revolutionary" nutrition and health findings. And isn't it marvelous how some magazines come up with a new twist on the "effortless diet" every month. Sure, it's all part of marketing, but how is one to know what to believe?

It's difficult for the professional, let alone the public, to keep up to date. The consumer also has a problem figuring out *whom* to believe.

While scanning the pages of an airline magazine on a recent trip, I found no less than five advertisements for companies selling college degrees—master's and doctorate, no less—through the mail. The highly touted electronic highway now allows modem-minded folks to get similar advanced degrees through the Internet. In almost all these cases, no classroom attendance is required. These "institutions give you credit for "life experience," and they charge a hefty tariff to dispense your diploma. One classic tale involves a scientist who was able to purchase a Ph.D. for his dog!

The downside to all these sheepskin shenanigans is that there are a number of folks calling themselves "doctor" without the necessary training. And what's more, their numbers will continue to increase.

Many questionable products will boast that the individual in charge is a "doctor" without revealing what type of doctor he or she is. It may be claimed that the "doctor" is "internationally known," or a "leading expert," but you should ask "Known by whom?" and "Where, exactly is he or she leading people?"

Be a skeptic and you can avoid being taken. There are a number of ways that questionable products can be foisted upon the public.

One common strategy is to use a collection of convincing true-to-life testimonials. The pitch follows the line that "it worked for them, so why not for you?" When you add in the support of someone with pseudo-credentials, you can end up with impressive marketing clout.

Another conduit for questionable products is the burgeoning field of multilevel marketing (MLM). This marketing technique has neighbor selling to neighbor, often trying to recruit them into their sales force. Many initial contacts for MLM sales are made through e-mail. I've found that when health-related products are being offered, the facts tend to take a back seat. In many cases the dealer has no real training in the health-related field.

Finally, just because something is new and different does not mean that it is nonsense. Often, progress in medicine and nutrition begins with ideas that are considered radical. The difference, however, comes in how the proponent proceeds. The scientist takes the new ideas to the laboratory for testing and evaluation. The charlatan goes directly to the public in search of financial gain.

Guidelines for Combating Health Fraud

- Make sure that the people giving you advice know what they're talking about. If they pass themselves off as experts, find out if this is the case.
- If your instincts tell you something is not right, or you are simply curious about their training, politely ask, ask, and then ask some more.
- If they cite training at an institution you have never heard of, consult a reference book, such as *College Degrees by Mail,* now in its 11th edition, by Berkeley resident John Bear, Ph.D. (Ten Speed Press, $12.95). This valuable book, which makes interesting reading in its own right, is an eye-opening look at the wide variety of institutions offering nontraditional degrees. (Bear's Ph.D., by the way, is from Michigan State University.)
- If you ever uncover health fraud, report it immediately. In the white pages of most phone books, under Consumer Complaint and Protection Coordinators, is a list of numbers you can use to contact the oversight agencies for most of the professional areas. You might also seek help from the media; there are many television and radio stations that have consumer reporters just itching to turn the tables on fraud in your town.

It's deceitful to claim expertise without training. And when the practice involves a health-related area, it can be downright dangerous. As there is no efficient way to purge all health areas of fraudulent practitioners, it always falls upon the consumer to be alert.

25. An Eating Plan
You Can Live With

The Need for a Unified Approach

We need to look at the connection between diet, health, and disease through one set of glasses. This tends to be difficult because today's age of scientific specialization overwhelms most chances for such a holistic view.

Consider, for instance, that the American Heart Association and one set of research scientists are focused on heart disease, while the American Cancer Society and a separate set of health scientists have their glasses trained on "the big C." Each group has their own set of scientific societies, journals, and professional meetings where research about "their" disease gets discussed.

No one would question that heart disease and cancer are different diseases—especially where treatment is concerned. For this reason, some specialization is essential. But if you looked at these diseases only from the standpoint of their dietary prevention programs, you couldn't tell them apart. Both heart disease and cancer recommend a reduction of dietary fat and an increase of the daily intake of vegetables, fruits, and grains. And by strange coincidence, the same eating plan is recommended to stave off arthritis, obesity, diabetes, and hypertension.

Clues from Our Eating History

You can get further testimony to the healthfulness of such an eating plan by examining our nutritional history. About 90 percent of the time we've been on this planet, our diet was high in fiber and low in fat. It wasn't until the last two hundred years, following the Industrial Revolution, that the American and Northern European diet began its shift toward higher levels of fat and lower fiber.

Although the palate was quick to embrace this change, our bodies apparently haven't had the same success. Research points to the earlier mode of consumption—lower fat, higher in vegetables, fruits, and grains—as the best way to avoid heart disease and cancer, now the top two killer diseases. In countries of Africa and Asia, where a change in diet never occurred, these diseases are almost nonexistent. Undoubtedly, there are other factors involved, but the connection between diet and disease cannot be ignored.

What is it about such a dietary change that could make it such a boon to health? The fact that the same type of diet is associated with a lower incidence of such a variety of maladies suggests that these diseases share something in common.

But rather than delving into complex scientific details, another way to look at it is that a greater emphasis on vegetables, fruits, and grains keeps the body in good health, and it's this higher state of health that fortifies the body's defenses against *all* diseases.

Picture it this way . . .

- In order for a disease to set up shop in a body, it has to find its way to the door, break down the lock, go inside, and then overcome the body's defensive guards that are primed to fight.
- When your diet has high levels of fat and you don't give

your body the nutrients it needs, you have essentially lit the path, unlocked the door, and sent the guard away.

What comes in that open door will reflect your genetic makeup and lifestyle. We cannot pick our parents, so we have to be cognizant of our health heritage. For example, if you're a smoker, lung cancer will likely be the first in line. If heart disease, colon, or breast cancer runs in your family, you have to be aware that there's a tendency for them to be at the head of the line.

Likewise, good health care and early diagnosis could make the difference between nipping a potentially serious problem in the bud or inadvertently allowing it to fester past any hope of recovery.

If you look at countries where they eat higher levels of fat *and* enjoy a good state of health, the cuisine also includes a high intake of grains, fruits, and vegetables. In the United States, our fat intake is high, but our intake of grains, fruits, and vegetables is only a fraction of what it needs to be.

In this country we continue to leave ourselves wide open for problems.

So Why Don't More of Us Eat Healthfully?

One answer might be the difficulty in making the connection between eating habits and long-term health. To be sure, those imperiled by a brush with heart disease or other diet-related malady can take to a new diet with religious fervor. But many heading down that same road are seemingly oblivious to constant reminders that a similar fate lies ahead.

Another potential problem could be misconceptions about what dietary change involves. Current guidelines state we should have no more than 30 percent of our Calories as fat. However, in a survey conducted by the American

Dietetic Association, fewer than 7 percent knew how to apply that number to their food selection.

Finally, it's important to understand that a good diet cannot guarantee health. But, all things being equal, a daily dose of health-promoting nutrients would have to be considered one of the most effective unified approaches to fighting disease. Having a diet based on grain, vegetables, and fruits is an excellent way to accomplish this.

An Eating Plan You Can Live With—
Making Health Happen

Basic Principles

- Principle Number One: Good nutrition does not involve a sacrifice in flavor.
- Your diet should include all the food groups, but the foundation of your eating plan should be nutrient-rich grains, vegetables, and fruits. Aim for a minimum of five servings a day of fruits and vegetables—the fresher the better. (A typical serving is a medium piece of fruit, 1 cup of a leafy vegetable, $1/2$ cup of fruit or cooked vegetables, $1/4$ cup of dried fruit, or 6 ounces of a fruit or vegetable juice.)
- An average figure for fat is about 20 to 30 percent of calories, *but* diets that are high in fruits, vegetables, legumes and whole grains, fish, nuts, and low-fat dairy products need not be restricted in terms of total fat so long as there is not an excess of calories.
- You don't have to include animal-based foods (meat, poultry, fish, dairy) to have a healthful diet. But, on the other hand, having these foods is not incompatible with health as long as you don't overdo it.
- Emphasize vegetable oils (predominantly monounsaturated) such as olive oil and canola oil.

- Keep your intake of partially hydrogenated fats to an absolute minimum. (Partial hydrogenation is the process by which liquid vegetable oils are hardened into semi-solid fats for use in processed food and fast-food frying. These oils have adverse effects and offer no counterbalancing nutritional benefits.)
- Everything you eat does not have to be bursting with good nutrition. You can enjoy most foods, as long as you follow the principles of balance, variety, and moderation.
- Embrace the idea that there are healthful approaches to food and approaches that are self-defeating and poorly balanced. You *can* have it all as long as you give your body the nutrient-rich foods it needs.

Food Planning, Preparation, and Serving

- Emphasize variety and moderation.
- When planning meals, keep in mind that soups are an excellent way to add flavors and fullness with a minimum of fat.
- When shopping for meat, purchase lower fat cuts and always trim visible fat before cooking.
- Have no more than two 3-ounce servings of meat, poultry, or fish a day. Try to have fish on the menu at least twice a week. (A 3-ounce serving is about the size of a pack of playing cards.)
- Aim for at least one meatless (vegetarian) day a week.
- Broil, bake, roast, stir fry, or steam instead of deep-fat frying. When you bypass deep-fried foods, you not only make a significant dent in your fat intake, you avoid potentially harmful elements.
- In poultry, most of the fat is in or just under the skin. It's all right to cook poultry with the skin on, but remove the skin before eating.
- Cook stews and meat-containing soups in advance, so that there's enough time to cool the dish and skim off any excess fat before serving.

- Use olive oil instead of a spreadable fat for breads. If a spreadable fat is desired, consider butter, or make your own "soft" spread by mixing butter with a liquid, monounsaturated oil such as canola, or a light-flavored olive. If you are going to use margarine, choose a liquid or tub margarine—one that contains either no partially hydrogenated fat or lists it no higher than third on the ingredient statement.
- When at the table, practice portion control. Have high-bulk/low-fat foods (grains, vegetables, and fruits) at every meal. Remember—whenever you eat until you feel full, you've had too much—it takes as long as twenty minutes for the mind to realize that the stomach is full.

Simple Substitutions

- By using nutrient-rich foods in place of traditionally high-fat products, you can make significant dents in your fat/Calorie intake. For example, substituting 1 cup of skim milk for whole milk every day saves 23,000 Calories over a year's time (2% low-fat for whole milk saves 10,600 Calories).
- Snack on dried figs and apricots, pretzels, or cut-up vegetables instead of chips.
- Rely on fish or some leaner cuts of meat.

Snack Time

- Plan ahead for snacks. When you wait until you feel hunger pangs, or it's your scheduled break time, you put yourself at the mercy of convenience foods that often are devoid of nutritional value and high in partially hydrogenated fats. At home and work, have a supply of fruits and cut-up raw vegetables, such as carrots and celery, in the refrigerator. Dried fruits, pretzels, or air-popped corn can also provide a satisfying treat.

Other Factors

- **Activity is the foundation of good health.** Even if you haven't the time or inclination for a regular exercise program, you should be able to find something that fits your lifestyle. Studies show that even when activity is at moderate levels—such as a brisk daily walk—there can be a significant payoff in better health.
- Drink at least eight glasses of water a day.
- Learn how to read the food label (consult chapter 18). This tool can help you choose between comparable products and assure that you get the most nutrition for your money.

Daily Nutritional Checklist

Here's a list of the healthiest and most nutrient-dense foods in every food category. It's designed to help you select the best foods for your daily menu. (*Note:* Some of the fruits and vegetables may not be available in all areas.) *There is also a list of fats and oils, listed in order of preference.*

VEGETABLE GROUP
3–5 SERVINGS

(A serving equals 1 cup raw leafy greens, or ¹/₂ cup cooked or chopped vegetables.)

Cooking & Salad greens (turnip, mustard, beet, collard, kale, romaine, leaf lettuce, parsley, arugula, amaranth, spinach)
Potatoes (white & sweet)
Corn (fresh & air-popped)
Leeks
Winter Squash
Carrots
Cabbage
Cauliflower

Asparagus
Red Peppers
Broccoli

DAIRY GROUP
2–3 SERVINGS

---

*(A serving equals 1 cup milk or yogurt, 1¹/₂ oz.
natural cheese, or 2 oz. processed cheese.)*

Skim Milk
1% Milk
Low-Fat Acidophilus Milk
Non-Fat Yogurt
Buttermilk
Sherbet
Fat-Free Frozen Desserts
Low-Fat Frozen Desserts
Reduced-Fat Cheese (fat-free, low-fat, or dry-curd)

BREADS, CEREALS, & GRAINS
6–11 SERVINGS

---

*(A serving equals 1 slice of bread, 1 cup dry cereal, or
¹/₂ cup cooked cereal, rice, or pasta.)*

Grains & Flours (barley, oats, buckwheat, rye, bulgur, mil-
let, quinoa, amaranth, flaxseed)
Hot or Cold Cereals
Bread (whole-wheat is best)
Pasta (whole-wheat is best)
Rice (brown is best)
Wheat Germ
Bran (wheat, rice, oat)
Baked Goods (bagels, pita bread, corn tortillas, matzos,
rice cakes, pretzels)

FRUIT GROUP
2–4 SERVINGS

(A serving equals a medium apple or orange, $1/4$ melon or grapefruit, $1/4$ cup dried fruit, or 1 cup berries.)

Bananas
Citrus (orange, grapefruit, lemon, lime)
Melons (cantaloupe, honeydew)
Black Currants
Berries (blackberries, raspberries, strawberries)
Tropical Fruits (papaya, guava, mango)
Kiwi
Dried Fruits (figs, apricots, prunes, dates)
Apples

PROTEIN GROUP:
MEAT, POULTRY, FISH, LEGUMES, EGGS, & NUTS
2–3 SERVINGS

(A serving of meat, fish, or poultry is about 3 oz.; a serving of legumes equals $1/2$ cup cooked beans; a serving of tofu is 4 oz.; a serving of nuts is 1 oz.)

Fresh Fish
Canned Fish (water pack)
Pork Tenderloin
Chicken (without skin)
Turkey (without skin)
Beef Top or Eye of Round
Egg Whites
Beans (pinto, navy, lima, garbanzo, kidney)
Black-eyed Peas, Lentils
Almonds, Walnuts, Pecans, Peanuts

FATS & OILS
No specific serving requirement

(A serving equals 1 tsp. oil or a spreadable fat, 1 tbsp. oil-based dressing.)

Preferred Oils: olive, canola, almond, safflower, sunflower, walnut, corn, sesame, peanut, cottonseed
Choose less often: butter, chicken fat, lard, palm kernel oil, coconut oil, liquid margarine, tub margarine
Choose rarely: vegetable shortening, stick margarine

WINE/ALCOHOL

If consumed, have no more than 1–2 drinks a day
(A drink is defined as 4 oz. wine, 12 oz. beer, or 1 oz. hard liquor.)

Glossary of Nutritional Terms

Absorption: The act of taking nutrients into the cells of the intestines.

Additives: Substances added to food.

Amino Acid: The basic building block of protein. Our body has about twenty-two different amino acids in its proteins.

Amylase: An enzyme produced by the pancreas that breaks carbohydrates into maltose, a double sugar made up of two glucoses attached to each other.

Anemia: A condition in which there is an inadequate number of red blood cells, which are the oxygen-carrying cells of the blood.

Antioxidant: A substance that prevents another substance from combining with oxygen.

Basal Metabolic Rate (BMR): The rate of energy (expressed in Calories) used when the body is at rest to keep the body processes such as breathing and heart rate going.

Bile: A substance produced by the liver and stored in the gall bladder, that is used during digestion to help emulsify fats and make them more receptive to the action of lipase.

Bioavailability: The extent to which a substance present in a food is available for absorption.

Body Mass Index (BMI): An index of weight in relation to height. It is equal to the weight in kilograms divided by the square of one's height in meters.

Calorie: A unit of energy, used to describe the energy value of foods.

Complementary Protein: Two proteins with amino acid profiles that complement each other, the combination of the two making a complete protein.

Complete Protein: A protein that contains all the essential amino acids.

Enzyme: Protein chemicals that act on foods, breaking them into their constituent parts. Each enzyme works in a specific way on only one type of food. For example, the enzyme that breaks complex carbohydrates into smaller carbohydrates has no effect on either fats or protein.

Essential Amino Acid (EAA): An amino acid the body cannot synthesize on its own. Essential amino acids must be provided by the diet for the body to be able to manufacture proteins.

Essential Fatty Acid: A fatty acid the body cannot make on its own in sufficient amounts to satisfy its needs.

Fat: Fatty acids that are solid at room temperature—example: coconut oil, lard, shortening.

Fatty Acid: The basic chemical structure of fats and oils.

Food Allergy: An adverse reaction to a food that involves the immune system.

Food Intolerance: An adverse reaction to a food that does not involve the immune system.

Fortification: The addition of nutrients to a food at levels that were not originally present in that food.

Hydrogenation: A high-pressure process that adds hydrogen to unsaturated fatty acids to make them more saturated. It is also called "hardening." During partial hydrogenation, some of the unsaturated fatty acids are changed into trans fatty acids.

Lipase: An enzyme produced by the pancreas that breaks down triglycerides into fatty acids and glycerol (the backbone to which the fatty acids are attached).

Lipid: A family that includes fats, oils, fatty acids, steroids, phospholipids, waxes, sterols (cholesterol), and triglycerides.

Lipoprotein: A protein–lipid combination specially adapted to carry lipids (i.e., triglycerides and cholesterol) around the body's water-based circulatory system.

Monounsaturated Fatty Acid: A fatty acid in which one pair of carbons has formed a double bond—example: oleic acid, found predominantly in olive and canola oils.

Oil: Fatty acids that are liquid at room temperature—example: corn oil.

Pasteurization: The process of heating milk or some other beverage in a way that kills the great majority of bacteria and disease-carrying microorganisms. It is not the same as sterilization, in which all microorganisms are killed.

Pepsin: An enzyme formed in the stomach that breaks down peptides into di-peptides (two amino acids).

Peptidase: An enzyme that breaks di-peptides into amino acids.

Peptide: A compound made from two or more amino acids.

Polyunsaturated Fatty Acid: A fatty acid in which there are at least two double bonds.

Protease: An enzyme produced by the pancreas that breaks large proteins into peptides.

Ptyalin: An enzyme present in the saliva (also called salivary amylase) that helps break large carbohydrates down into smaller ones.

Rennin: An enzyme in the gastric juice that curdles milk to ease its digestion. This is not to be confused with renin (one "n"), a kidney enzyme that plays a role in blood pressure.

Saturated Fatty Acid: A fatty acid that does not contain any double bonds between the carbon atoms.

Trans Fatty Acid: A type of unsaturated fatty acid in

which the double bond between two of the carbon atoms is less flexible than the standard cis type of bond. Trans fatty acids are usually produced through the process of partial hydrogenation.

Triglyceride: The most common form taken by fats and oil, in which three fatty acids are attached to a backbone, somewhat akin to the letter *E*.

Unsaturated Fatty Acid: A fatty acid that contains at least one double bond between a pair of carbon atoms.

Index